AF566987

Imaging in Esthetic Dentistry

Imaging in Esthetic Dentistry

Cary E. Goldstein, DMD

Private Practice
Atlanta, Georgia

Clinical Instructor of Oral Rehabilitation
Medical College of Georgia School of Dentistry, Augusta

Ronald E. Goldstein, DDS

Clinical Professor of Oral Rehabilitation
Medical College of Georgia School of Dentistry, Augusta

Adjunct Clinical Professor of Prosthodontics
Boston University Henry M. Goldman School of Dental Medicine

Adjunct Professor of Restorative Dentistry
The University of Texas Health Science Center at San Antonio

Visiting Professor
Department of Oral and Maxillofacial Imaging and Continuing Education
University of Southern California School of Dentistry, Los Angeles

David A. Garber, DMD

Clinical Professor of Periodontics
Clinical Professor of Oral Rehabilitation
Medical College of Georgia School of Dentistry, Augusta

Visiting Professor
Department of Prosthodontics
Louisiana State University

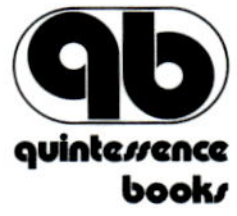

Quintessence Publishing Co, Inc

Chicago, Berlin, London, Tokyo, Paris, Barcelona,
São Paulo, Moscow, Prague, and Warsaw

To the two most important people in my life, my wife, Jody, and our son, Maxwell. — CEG

Dedicated to my wife, Judy, and my children, Cathy, Ken, and Rick. — REG

Ongoing thanks to my wife, Barbara, and my children, Karen, Jennifer, and Mike. — DAG

Library of Congress Cataloging-in-Publication Data

Goldstein, Cary E.
Imaging in Esthetic Dentistry / Cary E. Goldstein, Ronald E. Goldstein, David A. Garber.
p. cm.
Includes bibliographical references and index.
ISBN 0-86715-238-9
1. Dentistry—Aesthetic aspects. 2. Image processing—Digital techniques. 3. Dental photography. I. Goldstein, Ronald E. II. Garber, David A. III. Title.
[DNLM: 1. Esthetics, Dental. 2. Image Processing, Computer- Assisted WU 100 G6237e 1998]
RK54.G638—dc21
DNLM/DLC
for Library of Congress 97-39481
CIP

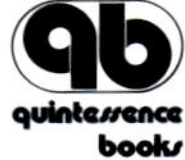

Published by Quintessence Publishing Co, Inc
551 N. Kimberly Dr.
Carol Stream, IL 60188

Printed in Hong Kong

Contents

Contributors

David Gane, DDS, BSc
President
Source Dental Image Inc.
White Rock, British Columbia
Canada

Arlen Lackey, DDS
Private Practice
Pacific Grove, California

Jonathan Levine, DMD
Private Practice
New York, New York

Wayne Rees
Vice President
Source Dental Image Inc.
White Rock, British Columbia
Canada

Barbara Wagner, RDH
Atlanta, Georgia

Edwin Zinman, DDS, JD
San Francisco, California

Special Contributors

Susan Hodgson, RDH
Atlanta, Georgia

Tony Scott
Indianapolis, Indiana

Foreword

The philosopher Santayana said that "beauty is pleasure objectified"—the physical embodiment of a mental concept . . . and therein lies the problem. When a patient has a mental concept of what a desired result might be—how is the dentist to objectify that concept of beauty? The answer, of course, is through imaging. Imaging in dentistry is finally maturing and is being recognized for its value in enhancing communication and clarifying concepts. A textbook for imaging is, then, a natural result of this maturation and recognition.

Dentists have come to accept the fact that an intraoral camera is a useful adjunct in modern practice, and patients expect to find an intraoral camera in the modern dental office. The problem has been that very few dentists have learned to use a camera to its optimum advantage, and to use imaging to define the mutual goals of both the patient and the dentist. It is much easier to obtain equipment than it is to receive competent, effective instruction, and make effective use of electronic adjuncts. This book provides a much needed reference for the dentist who wishes to make optimum use of an imaging system. For those who have yet to make such a purchase, the reasons for doing so should be overwhelming. The text complements the numerous illustrations—and it is the illustrations that do what text is unable to do—convey reality without ambiguity.

Multi-ethnic, multi-cultural practices bring many challenges to dentists wishing to provide esthetic services to their patients. It is especially in these circumstances that communication must be established, for what is esthetic in one culture is ugly in another. Dentists must remove their ego and communicate—not converse. This book provides real-world instruction of how to communicate, innovate, and create the best esthetic result for the particular patient being treated.

The greatest wish of a mentor is to be surpassed by his students. My compliments to Dr. Cary Goldstein in co-authoring the first comprehensive text on electronic imaging. It is a book to be studied and kept available for ready reference. No other medium does what this text accomplishes—the total rationale and technique for routinely incorporating electronic imaging into every dental practice.

Jack Preston, DDS

Preface

What began as a fascinating feature at the local department store's cosmetic counter has evolved into an indispensable part of the beauty industry, especially the esthetic dentist's armamentarium. Computer imaging takes human communication to a higher level of understanding and accuracy. When concepts and opinions are vague or limited by language, this technology complements a patient's spoken desires and is often the key to successful treatment decisions.

Every year billions of dollars are spent by dental consumers seeking to improve the appearance of their mouths from the failed efforts of well-meaning dentists. Often it is not the disappointment of unmet spoken desires, but *unspoken* expectations. The sad and surprising truth is that most of these poor results could have been avoided through the use of computer imaging prior to treatment.

For example, at what point is a tooth too long or too short to be esthetically pleasing? This can be determined by visualizing different tooth lengths "in the patient's mouth" on the monitor. Imaging has the potential to save much time and expense by reducing the occurrence of failure.

Although it may have begun as a communication tool, computer imaging is increasingly becoming an important diagnostic tool for dentists. It is just as important for the dentist to be able to know what may work well for a particular patient as well as what may *not* work. Even after the desired size and shape of a tooth has been given definition, imaging can give assurance that the desired tooth would comfortably fit in the mouth's anatomy and provide good function.

It would be difficult to practice esthetic restorative dentistry today without the use of the intraoral camera. A special inclusion in this book is a chapter focusing on its use. And while the intraoral camera enables the patient to see the problem, imaging takes the process a step further, helping the patient to visualize the potential solution as well. Computer imaging, whereby both patient and dentist view an image that has incorporated the desired esthetic improvements, is also a communication tool for other members of the dental team, including specialists and the dental laboratory technician who are both so integrally involved in achieving the desired results.

Computer imaging allows visualization of alternative treatment options, so patients can make informed choices that satisfy their needs. The patient thus becomes both co-diagnostician and co-therapist—from the early diagnostic phase through the various stages of treatment, placement of the final restoration, and even into the maintenance phase.

Finally, computer imaging allows not only the patient and his or her dentist to influence the treatment decision, but it allows the patient to incorporate other esthetic advisors—be it spouse, friends, or relatives—before final treatment decisions are made. The opportunity for this input has become a significant factor for increasing both the acceptance of treatment plans as well as post-treatment satisfaction.

This book was written for dentists and their auxiliaries who are actively seeking to improve their standard of patient satisfaction and considering adding computer imaging technology to their practice. Advice for the prepurchase stage is provided, as are step-by-step techniques and tips for initial use of imaging. This book is also for the experienced user who wants to expand and improve his or her technical imaging skills, as well as communication skills.

Computer imaging is not a gimmick; it is an invaluable part of both the communication and diagnostic aspects of esthetic treatment planning in dentistry. Those practitioners who have embraced the technology have experienced greater patient understanding, acceptance, and satisfaction with their treatment plans and results. We believe that this technology will one day be the rule rather than the exception in the esthetic dental practice. Its benefit to dentistry is simply too extensive to ignore.

Acknowledgments

We would like to express our gratitude to the many individuals who helped make this book possible. First and foremost, our contributors, who brought their expertise and knowledge to the text, deserve our utmost thanks.

The dental, esthetic, and technical consultants who helped pack these pages with pearls of information are David Cooper, Paul Davies White, Steven Seltzer, Dr. Paul Yurfest, Dr. Tony Levitas, Tom Greggs, Dr. Jack Preston, Dr. Ken Neuman, Dr. Peter Mills, Dr. Wally Dyer, Dr. Phil Knall, Dr. Woody Oakes, Dr. Arun Nayyar, and in particular Dr. Robert (Pete) Pickron, who first introduced us to the technology.

Barbara Wagner, RDH, imaged more than 80% of the cases presented here. This text would simply not be viable without her innovative imaging, authoring, and endless hours of communication with our patients and then recreating their smiles at her monitor.

A special word of thanks must be given to one of imaging's forefathers, Tony Scott. His invaluable contribution only begins to be described when we mention the sometimes 'round-the-clock time and energy he devoted to teaching us, as well as helping to develop our presentations of this technology.

We further acknowledge the contributions of the pioneers who developed esthetic imaging for cosmetology and plastic and reconstructive surgery. They paved the way for us.

These pages have been edited numerous times to update information, ensure accuracy, and improve readability. We thank Susan Hodgson, Sheila Lombardo, Enid Draluck, and Elliott Kanter. Clerical assistance was provided by Cynthia Clement, Margie Smith, Suzanne Peach, Tina Sjogren, and Candace Paetzhold. Our staffs have been behind us 100%; without them, we would not have been able to complete this book.

Two individuals, Dr. David Gane and Wayne Rees, deserve special recognition for their great help with all aspects of the project.

The Quest For Beauty

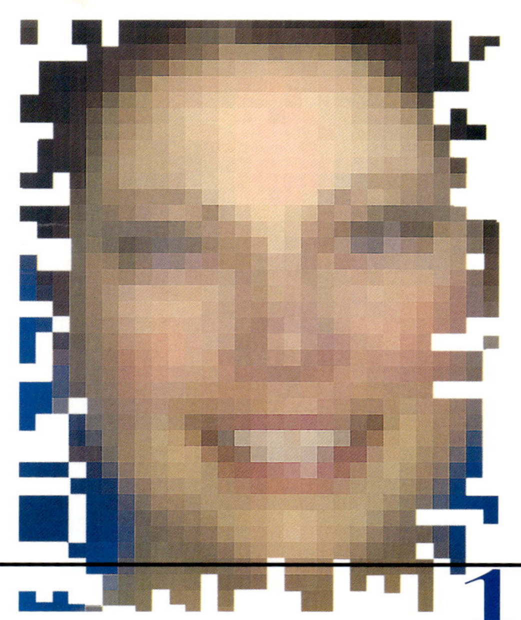

1

Beauty is that "which gives the highest degree of pleasure to the senses or to the mind and suggests that the object of delight approximates one's conception of an ideal."[1] Ever since primitive people first smeared their faces and bodies with pigments from the earth and admired the result, the quest for beauty has been expressed by every human culture.

Standards of Beauty

The human brain works much like a computer, storing information and recalling it at a later time. Standards for measuring beauty are actually a compilation and comparison of everything you have seen or experienced. When you look at a flower and think, "That's beautiful," in your mind's eye you are comparing your response to this flower in relative terms to every other flower you have seen. The same is true when you look at a smile.

Standards for measuring beauty are actually a compilation and comparison of everything you have seen or experienced.

It is true that standards of beauty change over time and across cultures. Members of some African tribes, for example, perforate their lips, ears, or noses in order to insert shells, colored stones, or gems. Among the Chinese nobility, the tiny bound feet of females were an important standard of beauty and status. Classical cultures of Greece and Rome based their standards of beauty on set rules of proportion and composition.[2]

While the various cultures of the world, past and present, may differ widely in their standards of beauty, the response to beauty is universal and spans all time.

The Response to Beauty

Psychologists have amassed considerable evidence that society places a great amount of importance on appearance. Various studies show that attractive people have more success in obtaining everything from dates to jobs to favorable jury verdicts. A 1987 report by Langlois et al[3] found that infants respond more positively to attractive faces than to unattractive ones, and prefer faces with soft curves to those with sharp angles. Research also demonstrates that attractive men and women tend to have higher paying and more prestigious jobs. Criminologists report that good-looking criminals are treated more leniently by juries and, in general, are more likely to receive lighter sentences than their less attractive counterparts. Teachers tend to be less harsh when disciplining attractive children, while both students and teachers perceive good-looking children to be smarter and more likely to succeed. Thus, there should be no question that it is advantageous in our society for individuals to make every effort to optimize their appearance.[4]

Proportions of Beauty

Many factors influence the perception of beauty, including makeup, clothing, jewelry, and facial expressions. However, it is the *relational proportion* of our physical features that is the primary factor in determining the perception, conscious or subconscious, of beauty.

Cunningham attempted to mathematically assess physical beauty.[5] In a study rating the attractiveness of 50 females, more than half of whom were finalists in an international beauty pageant, he concluded that:

1. The width of an eye should be three-tenths that of the face as measured at eye level (Fig 1-1a)
2. The chin length should be one-fifth the total height of the face (Fig 1-1a)
3. The vertical distance from the center of the eye to the bottom of the eyebrow should be one-tenth the height of the face (Fig 1-1b)
4. The height of the visible eyeball should be one-fourteenth the height of the face (Fig 1-1b)
5. The total area of the nose should be less than five percent of the total area of the face (Fig 1-1c)
6. The ideal mouth is 50 percent of the width of the face measured at mouth level (Fig 1-1c)

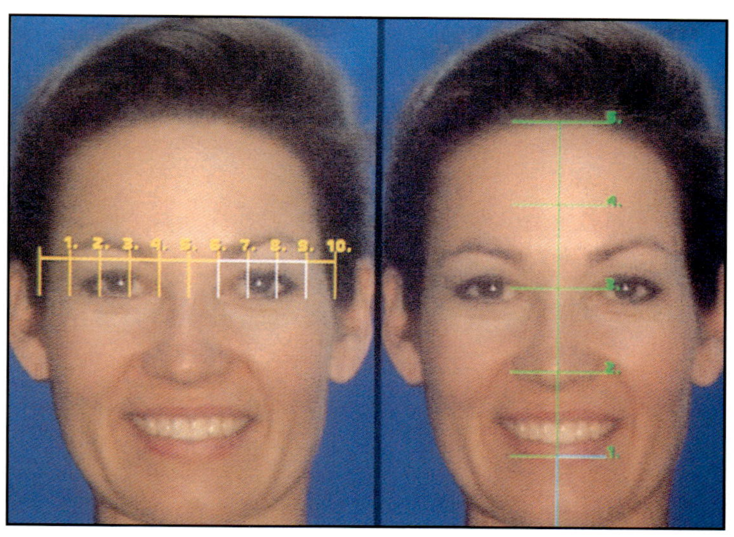

Fig 1-1a *Left, Eye width should be 3/10 the width of the face at eye level. Right, The chin should be 1/5 the height of the face. Figures 1-1a to 1-2 are based on Cunningham's five findings.*

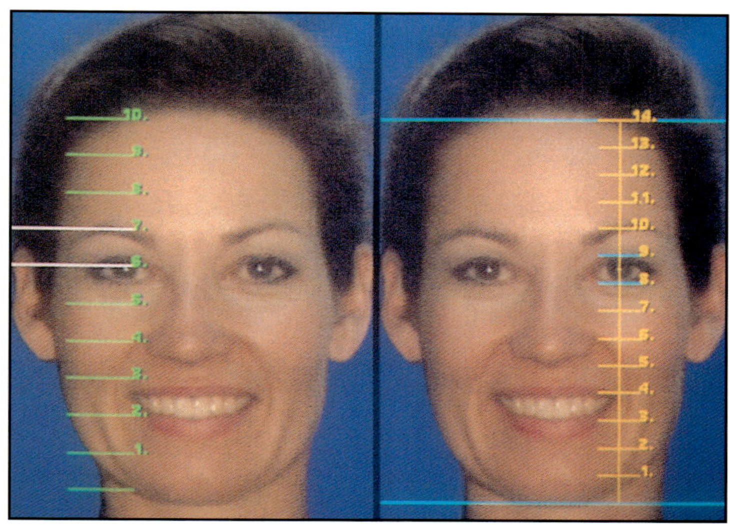

Fig 1-1b *Left, The vertical distance from the center of the eye to the bottom of the eyebrow should be 1/10 the height of the face. Right, The height of the visible eyeball should be 1/14 the height of the face.*

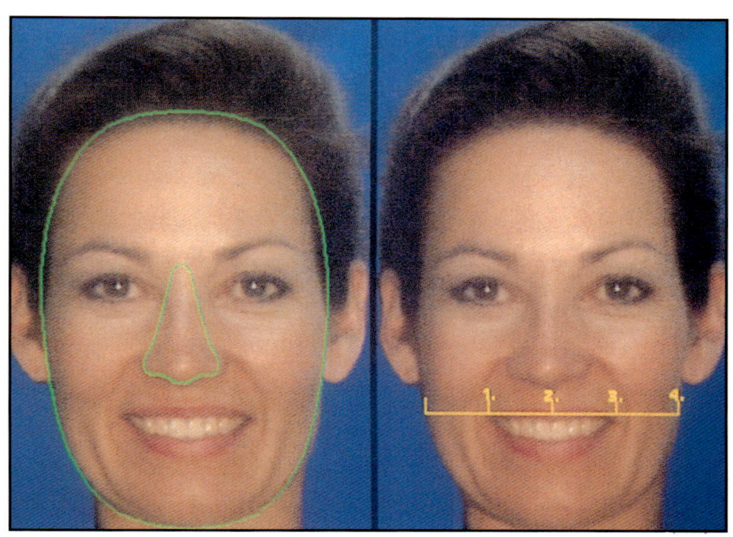

Fig 1-1c *Left, The total area of the nose should be less than 5% of the total area of the face. Right, The mouth should be 50% of the width of the face at mouth level.*

Cunningham's findings suggest that large eyes, a small nose and chin, high cheekbones, and a large, balanced smile are considered to be the physical attributes of a beautiful female face. Likewise, the handsome male face will have these same attributes but with the modifications of a relatively small nose, bushy eyebrows, and prominent chin (Fig 1-2).

These mathematical calculations reveal a harmony of proportion between features. When any one of these features is out of harmony, we tend to perceive that person as deviating from normal. If the features are brought into harmony and symmetry, the person is then viewed as attractive.

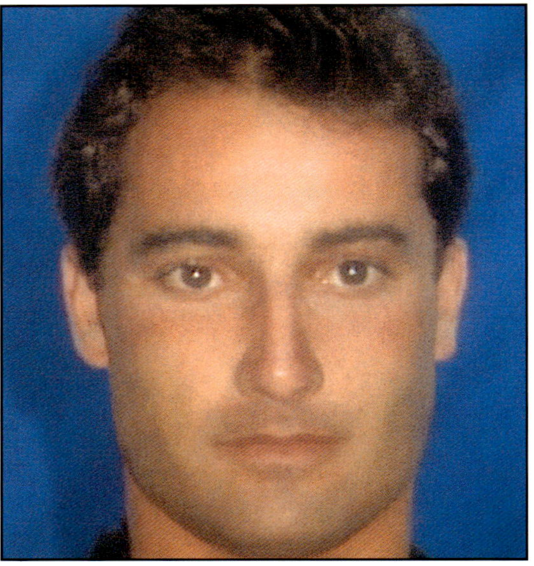

Fig 1-2 Cunningham's handsome male face.

Enhancing Beauty

We have many options available to alter and enhance our appearance, including cosmetic illusion through makeup and hairstyle, plastic and orthognathic surgery, as well as esthetic dentistry. When actual anatomical features cannot be changed, illusions can camouflage the lack of harmony. Women, for example, may use makeup to contour the cheeks and nose. Eyebrows can be arched to create the illusion of height, lips can be outlined larger or smaller, and the area around the eyes can be shadowed to appear larger and well spaced (Fig 1-3). In men, facial hair can be shaved or grown in various patterns. A beard can disguise a receding chin, and a mustache can conceal a long or unbalanced upper lip. False hair can be attached to the scalp to conceal baldness, and sideburns can be grown in various lengths to create the illusion of better facial form. These methods can play a major role in increasing one's self-confidence and promote self-esteem (Fig 1-4).

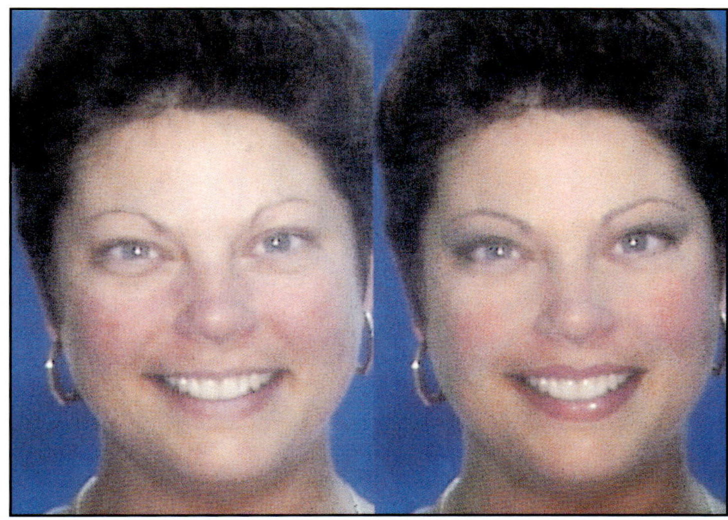

Fig 1-3 *Notice how the addition of makeup can create illusions of larger, well-spaced eyes, a more contoured face and nose, and larger lips.*

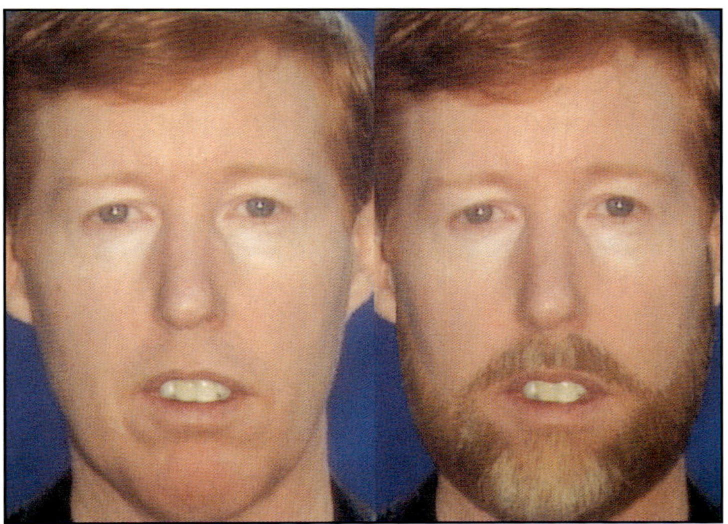

Fig 1-4 *Facial hair disguises a long lip and recessive chin in this man.*

Exercise and diet can often improve the shape of the body and, if that fails to produce the desired results, plastic surgery offers a variety of options. Liposuction can reduce fatty deposits in specific areas. Breasts can be augmented, reduced, or repositioned to improve esthetics. Plastic surgery can improve the relative proportions of the face, and therefore facial harmony, through procedures such as nasal reduction, chin and cheekbone augmentation, or elevation of eyebrows. Smiles can also be dramatically improved through orthodontics, bleaching, bonding, laminating, crowning, and other esthetic procedures.[6]

Alterations to improve appearance can result in positive changes in personality and self-esteem. Naturally, any cosmetic procedure should be undertaken with careful planning, realistic expectations, and a thorough understanding of the inherent risks and complications that can occur.

The quest for beauty is never ending and ever changing. Those who once had it want to restore it. Those who may never have experienced it may want to achieve it. And while relative standards may change, human nature ensures that people will continue to strive for the harmonious physical attributes that are so pleasing to the senses.

References

1. Webster's New World Dictionary of American English. Third College Edition. 1988.
2. Goldstein RE. Esthetics in Dentistry, ed 2, vol I. Toronto: Decker, 1998.
3. Langlois JH, Roggman LA, Casey RH, et al. Infant preferences for attractive faces: Rudiments of a stereotype? Dev Psychol 1987;23:363–369.
4. Goldstein RE. Esthetic dentistry—a health service? J Dent Res 1993;72:641–642.
5. Cunningham M. Measuring the physical in physical attractiveness: Quasi-experiments on the sociobiology of female facial beauty. J Pers Soc Psychol 1986;50: 925–935.
6. Goldstein RE. Change Your Smile, ed 3. Chicago: Quintessence, 1997.

Improving *Visualization* In Your Practice

2

When patients come to you for an esthetic consultation, you may readily visualize a variety of appropriate corrections and enhancements. Yet, can you be sure that you accurately communicate your visualization to each patient? Before the development of computer imaging technology, dentists relied on study casts, diagnostic wax-ups, markers, wax or composite mock-ups in the mouth, or pictures of other patients with similar problems and solutions. Unfortunately, in most situations, these aids are inadequate when patients must be able to comprehend accurately how any specific alteration will affect their appearance.

Unlike study casts and the other diagnostic tools ... computer imaging graphically illustrates proposed treatment options to each patient in a highly personalized form.

Complicating your communication challenge is the fact that most patients know little about the limits or potentials of esthetic dentistry, and they may have unrealistic ideas about what can or cannot be achieved. A young patient may want a "perfect" set of straight, even anterior teeth, not realizing that incisal edge wear is a characteristic of an older smile. Similarly, some patients may unconsciously expect receded gingival tissue to be remedied by a series of porcelain veneers. Such patients may be ultimately dissatisfied unless shown how periodontal surgery, orthodontics, or maxillofacial surgery can help achieve the best results.

Unlike study casts and the other diagnostic tools that are impersonal or imprecise, computer imaging graphically illustrates proposed treatment options to each patient in a highly personalized form using digitized pictures of them in before-and-after scenarios. Guesswork is transformed into true predictability that patients can see and accept.

Computer imaging can not only demonstrate the possible results of various treatment options, it can show patients how they may look during the interim stages of a lengthy or complex treatment process. Of additional importance is the ability to show patients what results cannot or *should not* be attempted, and to help them to understand and accept the esthetic reasons for your diagnosis.

One of the most exciting and valuable aspects of computer imaging is that it promotes proactive patient involvement in their treatment planning. It encourages them to express their likes and dislikes regarding alternate options and allows the opportunity for their creative feedback. Most importantly, you can learn exactly what their true expectations are and advise them if these expectations are unrealistic. Patients are then more likely to pursue the appropriate treatment and be satisfied with the result, as well as appreciate your efforts to achieve the best result possible.

The better you communicate with your patients, the greater the likelihood that you will please your patients. Computer imaging demonstrates to your patients that your practice utilizes state of the art technology that optimizes care and results. In one study, 92% of patients responding to a 1988 survey agreed that "computer imaging should be a routine part of preoperative cosmetic surgical evaluation."[1]

Advantages and Disadvantages of Traditional Visualization Aids

Traditional visualization aids have their limitations; in fact, some have more disadvantages than advantages.[2]

Study Casts

Probably the most often used and least expensive form of visualization aids are hand-articulated casts. These allow dentists and technicians to rapidly plan conventional restorative treatment prior to altering the teeth. Unfortunately, these casts have limited ability to demonstrate intended treatment to patients. In the absence of natural tooth color, the nuances of light and shadow, and the surrounding face, lips, and gingival soft tissue, study-cast teeth are out of context with the total esthetic picture (Fig 2-1).

Diagnostic Wax-up on Study Casts

Altering a study cast by sectioning and repositioning crowded or spaced teeth or contouring with or without the addition of wax to simulate an intended treatment plan is a typical way for dentists and technicians to communicate. The wax-up is an accurate method to measure and plan tooth proportion. While this is effective for dentist-laboratory communication, the diagnostic wax-up is an expensive and time-consuming procedure that, like the study cast, is not an effective tool for patient communication and visualization (Fig 2-2).

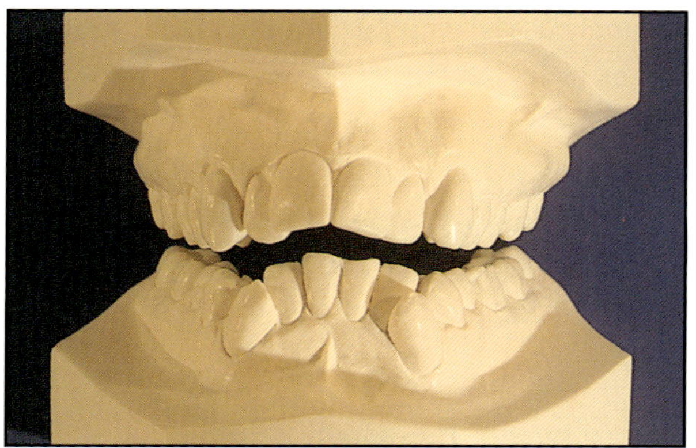

Fig 2-1 Many patients have difficulty envisioning the results of dental therapy without the framework of their lips and face.

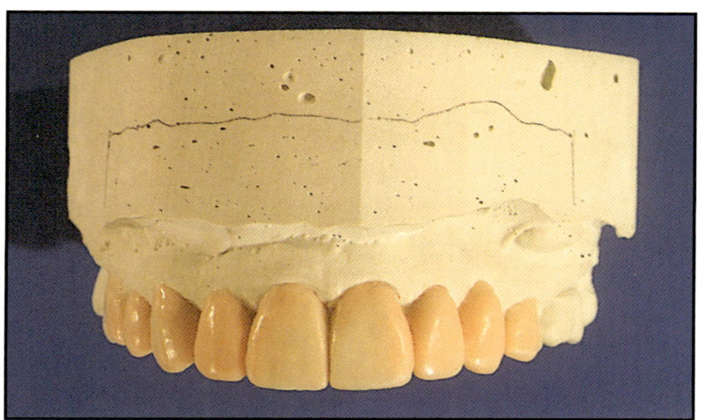

Fig 2-2 Even the best diagnostic wax-up may have yellow, blue, or green teeth, making it even more difficult for a patient to accurately visualize treatment outcomes.

Alcohol Markers

Alcohol markers offer a fast, simple, and inexpensive way to demonstrate minor changes in tooth form. Using a black marker on dry teeth, you can outline or mask areas to be removed. When standing about three feet from a mirror, your patient will be able to visualize the effects of cosmetic contouring as the black marker blends in with the darkness of the oral cavity behind the teeth. While this procedure is useful to simulate the removal of tooth structure, it is of no help in conveying the effects of other treatment modalities such as bonding or bleaching (Fig 2-3a and b).

Fig 2-3a and b The use of alcohol markers can help a patient visualize the results of cosmetic contouring.

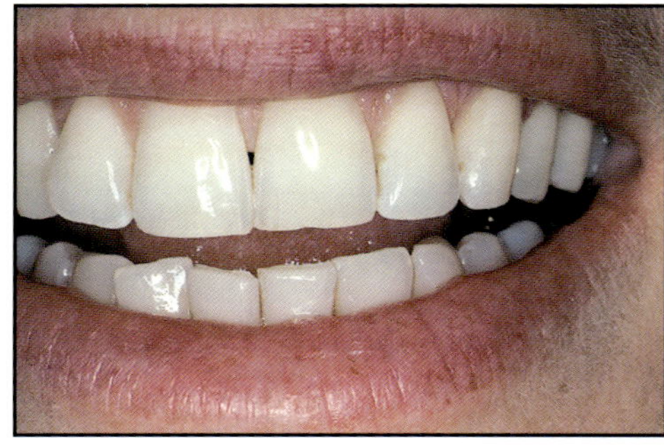

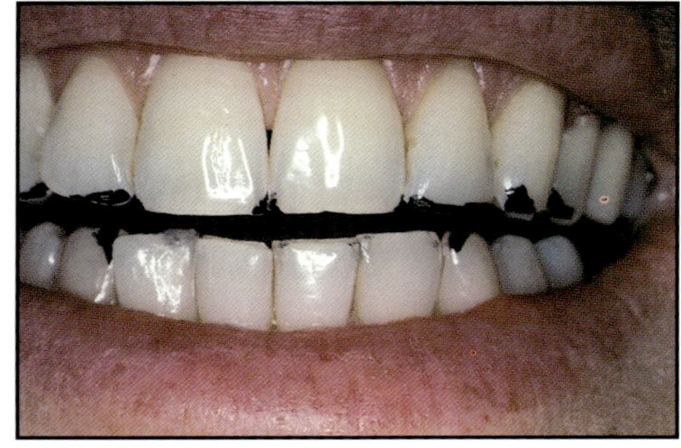

Photographs of Similar Patients

Another communication option is to show your patients photographs or drawings of other patients who have undergone procedures similar to those that you are recommending. This can help patients see the proposed result. The consumer book *Change Your Smile* was developed specifically to educate patients about the range of treatment options available and to offer visual examples of each alternative.[3] Although extremely useful when you want to raise your patients' esthetic dental IQ, as well as initiate the process of self diagnosis, it is only an educational beginning and not meant to take the place of seeing your proposed correction on your patient's own face. Photographs of someone else can be impersonal and may not sufficiently illustrate your patient's particular problem, making it difficult for them to adequately visualize how the proposed change can affect their appearance.

Direct Intraoral Simulation Using Wax or Composite Resin

When additions to teeth are needed, you can place a soft, tooth-colored wax or composite resin on the teeth and sculpt it to simulate proposed changes. However, this technique is time-consuming and is not effective for cosmetic contouring, periodontal procedures, or most orthodontic treatment plans (Fig 2-4).

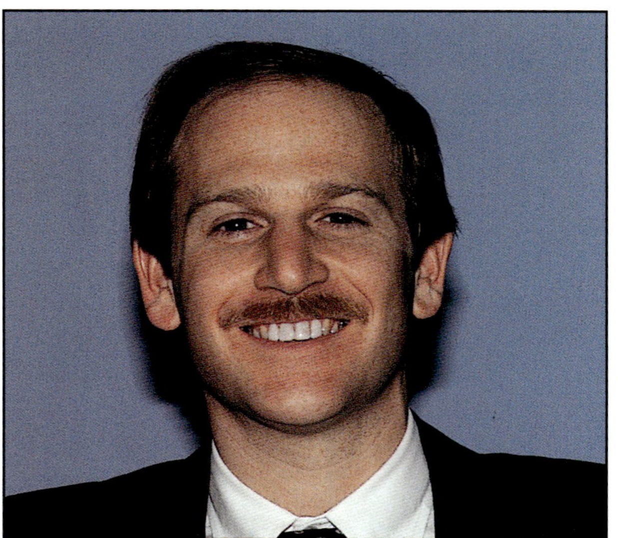

Fig 2-4 *White wax or composite placed and sculpted on the teeth is a step closer to true visualization for the patient.*

Vacuform Matrix and Composite Resin

Discerning patients who request a more personalized version of their projected esthetic result may require a more lifelike and detailed method of visualization. A useful technique is to fabricate a clear vacuform matrix formed over a cast of your patient's teeth. This is covered with tooth and/or tissue-colored materials, and fitted over your patient's existing teeth. These diagnostic prostheses can produce a realistic result and show many intended changes in tooth form, position, and color.

For patients with protruding anterior teeth, which may appear straight even though the whole arch is not in the intended position, this appliance may exacerbate the disfigurement and be counterproductive to the entire consultative process. Also, this technique is even more time-consuming and expensive than a diagnostic wax-up (Fig 2-5a to c). However, for exacting patients, these techniques can serve as a valuable adjunct in helping them to comprehend your intended esthetic changes.

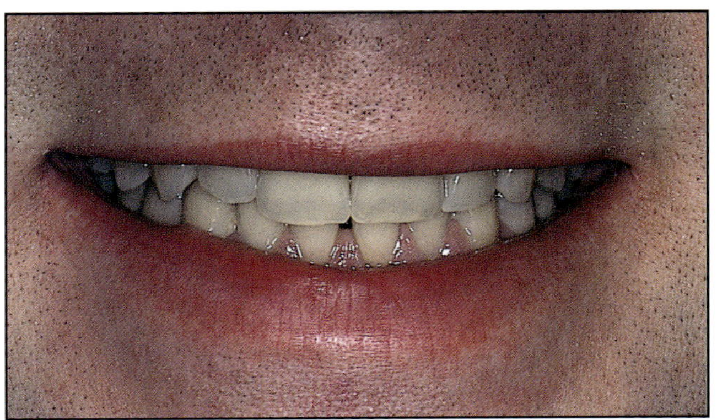

Fig 2-5a *This patient wanted to visualize himself with a larger, brighter smile.*

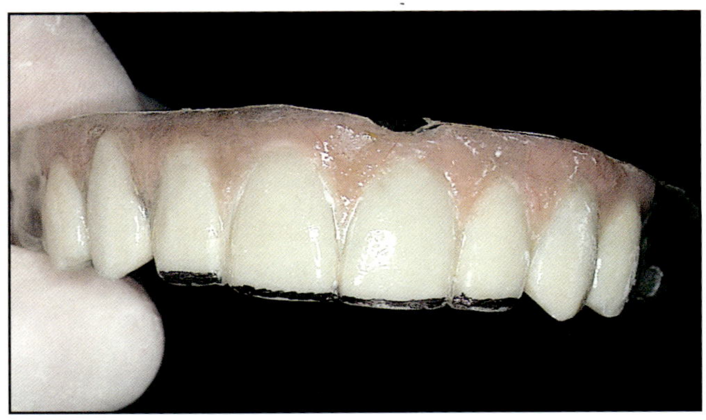

Fig 2-5b *A clear vacuform matrix was made to fit his arch. Tooth and gingiva-colored acrylics were added to the outside of the matrix to show the intended results.*

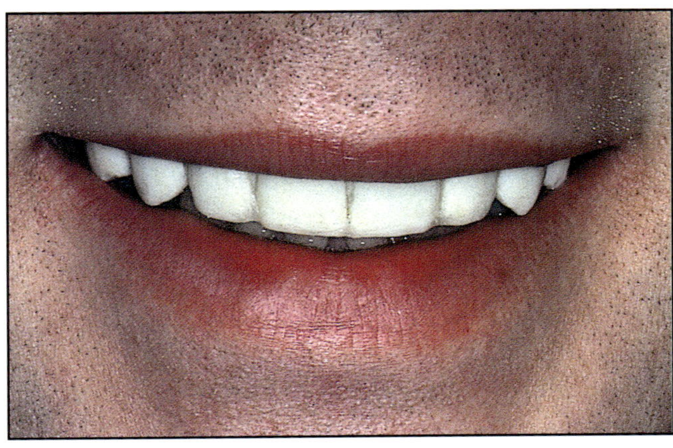

Fig 2-5c *The appliance in place shows the patient with the smile he wants.*

Combination Treatment Planning

Combining one or more of the previously discussed visualization techniques can aid in patient communication. The patient who presents with multiple problems, such as a maxillary anterior diastema, lower crowding, and a need for cosmetic contouring, may justify the extra time, effort, and expertise it will require for multiple visualization techniques. This might require closing the maxillary diastema with white wax or composite resin, building out the overlapped teeth with white wax or composite, and finally, using a black alcohol marker to create the illusion of contouring jagged or sharp line angles, shortening, or slenderizing the teeth.

Compared to the above diagnostic tools, the information gathered and presented in a diagnostic computer imaging evaluation is far superior. It is faster and more effective in demonstrating a variety of treatment options and selecting appropriate solutions that a patient can identify and apply to his or her situation.

Improving Lab Communication

Improved communication with outside laboratories for the fabrication of fixed prostheses is another advantage of computer imaging. Few dentists are fortunate enough to have an in-house laboratory and must instead rely on their ability to accurately communicate their needs to an outside dental laboratory technician. In most instances, the laboratory technician is guided solely by casts of the preparations, an opposing cast, bite registration, a prescription (with the patient's sex, age, and chosen shade), and sometimes a pretreatment study cast. Dentists and patients then expect to receive restorations from the laboratory that reflect what each has visualized. But as the public becomes more esthetically aware, dentists can no longer expect this to suffice. More information and alternative forms of communication will be needed to satisfy the subjective esthetic demands of the patient.

A simple photograph of the patient, with your interpretation of the appearance of the final restoration, can help the laboratory. When technicians are able to visualize the relative relationship of the teeth, lips, and gums within the patient's facial structure, the color of the existing teeth, and the smile, they are more apt to develop appropriate restorations. A computer-generated image of the patient showing the desired esthetic result, including tooth shape, relative color and contour of the teeth, and how these changes affect the dynamics of a smile, is even more effective (Fig 2-6).

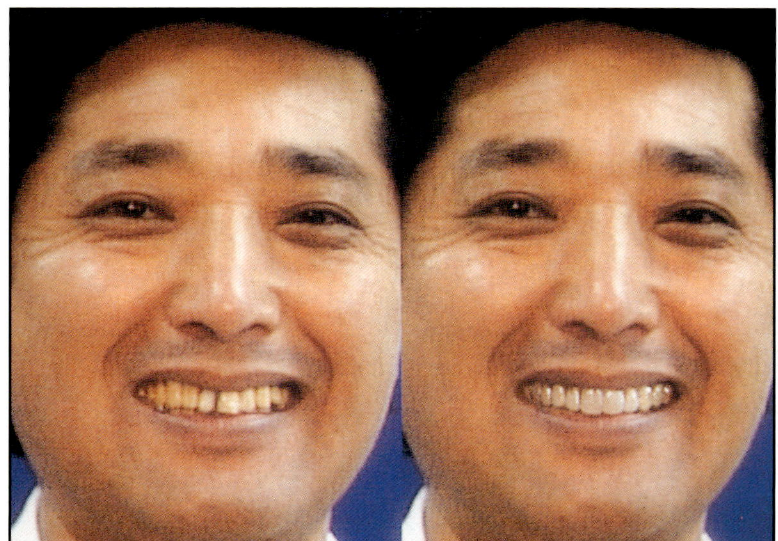

Fig 2-6 A before-and-after image of intended esthetic results may enhance your technician's ability to deliver superior prosthetics.

With a photograph, the shape and contour of the teeth, which may be more relevant to a successful result than the shade, can be copied by the technician. Equally important, an image can help the technician identify potential problems and limitations before attempting to fabricate the prosthetics. Any changes necessary to the preparations could then be made in advance, avoiding possible patient dissension and the extra expense of esthetic failure. In short, computer imaging has the potential to eliminate many costly and time-consuming mistakes and remakes.

References

1. Thomas JR, Freeman MS, Remmler DJ, Ehlert TK. Analysis of patient response to preoperative computerized video imaging. Arch Otolaryngol Head Neck Surg 1989;115:793–796.
2. Goldstein RE. Esthetics in Dentistry, ed 2, vol 1. Toronto: Decker, 1998.
3. Goldstein RE. Change Your Smile, ed 3. Chicago: Quintessence, 1997.

Further Reading

Goldstein CE, Goldstein RE, Garber DA. Computer imaging: an aid to treatment planning. J Calif Dent Assoc 1991;19;47–51.

Nathanson O. Dental imaging by a computer: a look at the future. JADA 1991; 122:45–46.

Golub-Evans J. Imaging helps induce balky patients, colleagues to accept best treatment. Dentist 1990;68:1–32.

The *Intraoral* Camera

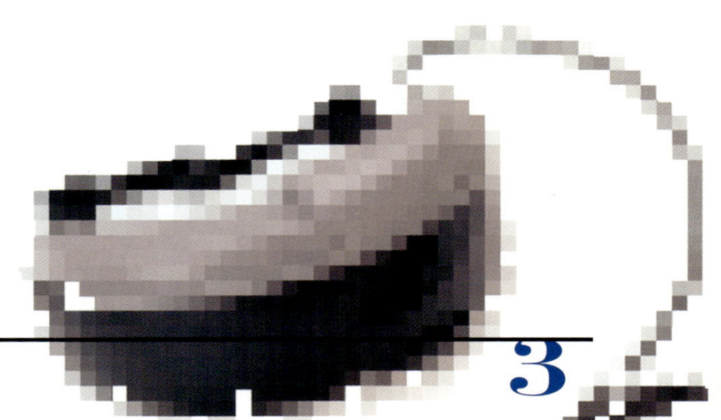

3

As patients become increasingly educated consumers, they expect to see the evidence of the problems you detect in their mouths. It isn't enough anymore to simply tell them that their teeth need to be restored. Fumbling attempts to have the patient focus on a hand-held mirror or your mouth mirror are inadequate for a progressive practice.

If your patient cannot see the problem, he or she often will not accept the solution.

With the aid of an intraoral camera, you can conduct a "tour" of the mouth (at 10 to 40 times life size), exploring and documenting the state of your patient's oral health. This can be especially helpful in new-patient interviews. Usually patients who change dentists will begin by scheduling a routine prophylaxis and checkup. In your initial examination, you may find numerous teeth in need of restoration or replacement—teeth that previous dentists may have "watched" for years. Understandably, your new patient could be shocked by what they could feel are your drastic findings. With an intraoral camera, however, you can show them the evidence. Your patients will be able to easily see the problems you find, such as worn-out, leaking, and defective amalgam restorations, decay, periodontal disease, or other pathologies (Fig 3-1a and b). If your patient cannot see the problem, he or she often will not accept the solution.

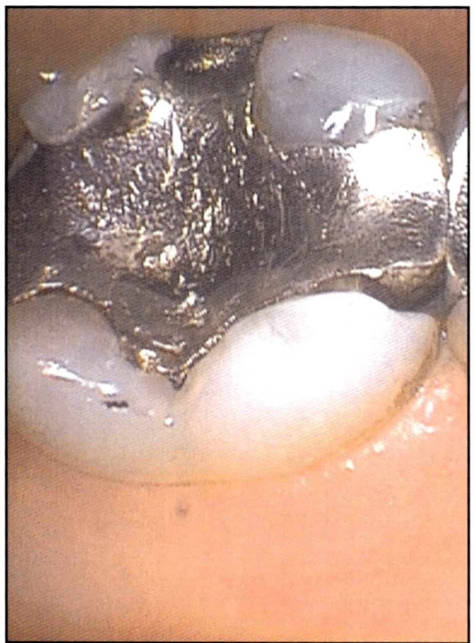

Fig 3-1a Your patient can easily see the defect in this restoration and the need for replacement.

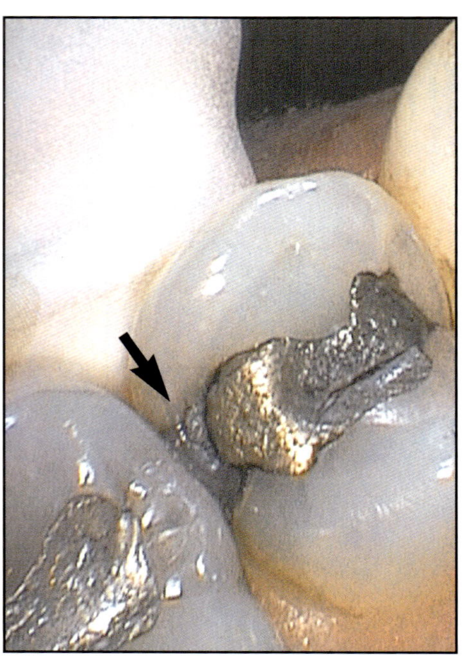

Fig 3-1b Decay is seen on this tooth.

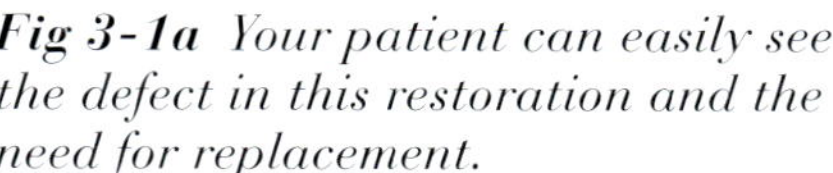

Common problems revealed by the intraoral camera

- Old, fractured, and tarnished amalgams (Fig 3-2)
- Leaking, stained, and fractured composites (Fig 3-3)
- Worn restorations
- Malposed, missing, or decayed teeth
- Microcracks with or without staining (Fig 3-4)
- Open margins
- Plaque and calculus (Fig 3-5)
- Periodontal problems
- Probing depths (Fig 3-6)
- Esthetic problems
- Tissue recession
- Tooth abrasion

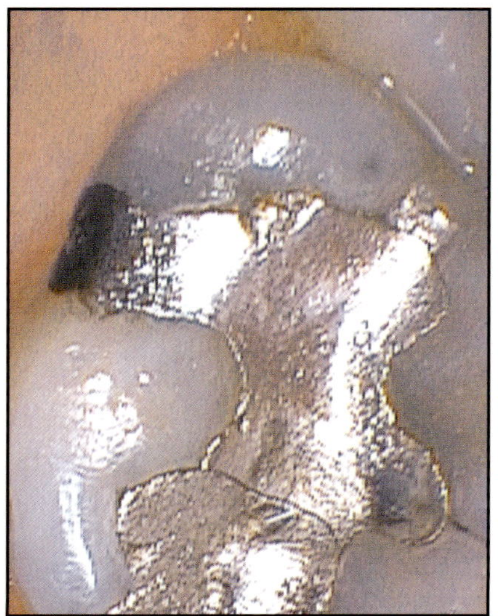

Fig 3-2 Fractured amalgam restorations can be easily diagnosed.

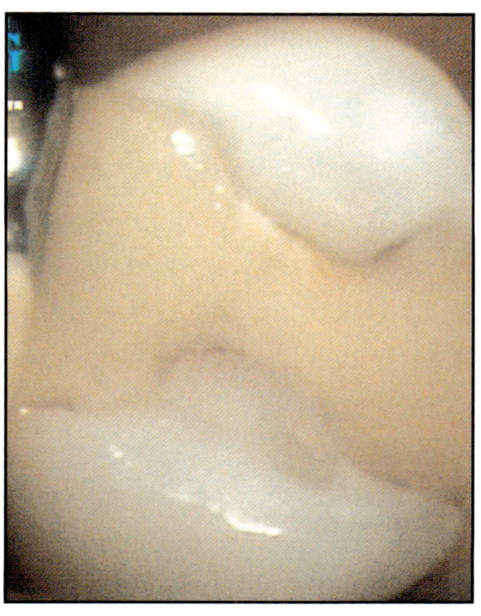

Fig 3-3 The intraoral camera shows your patient that this "white" filling is actually leaking.

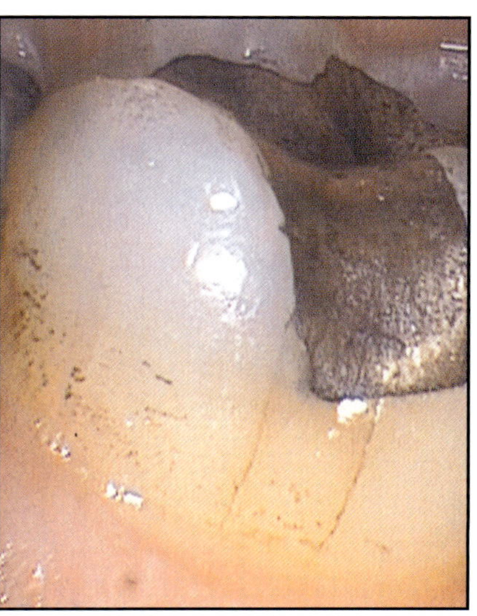

Fig 3-4 Microcracks often radiate from old amalgam restorations.

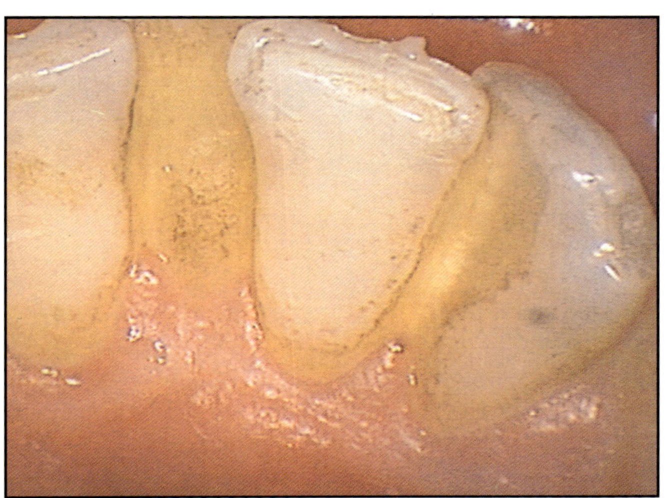

Fig 3-5 Patients can now see the calculus buildup on the lingual aspects of their lower anterior incisors.

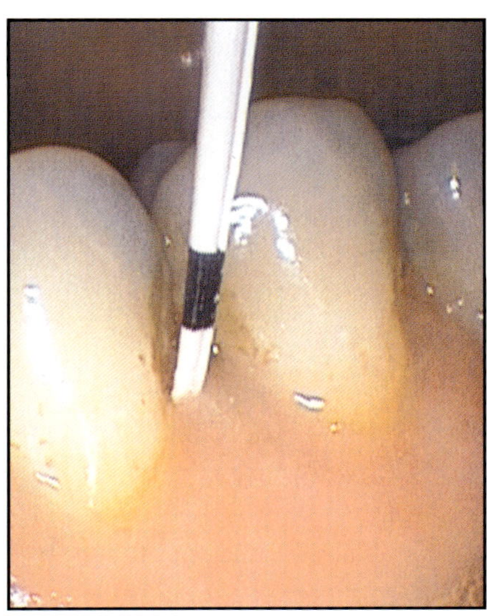

Fig 3-6 Showing a patient how deeply a probe penetrates their sulcus is an excellent use of the camera.

The intraoral camera is similarly useful with established recall patients. You should show these patients areas that you have been watching that now require treatment. You also can point out the healthy areas that may have improved as a result of either your therapy or their home care. Thus, the intraoral camera is a powerful and positive method to motivate patients to continue regularly scheduled maintenance. Conversely, if their situation is unsatisfactory or deteriorating, your patient can see the need for further treatment and/or increased home care. This allows your patient to become a "co–decision maker": he or she decides with you to treat the problem now, before it becomes larger or impossible. This is conservative esthetic dentistry at its optimal level. At this point "recalls" can become "interventions," an opportunity that educated patients will be reluctant to miss.

Although you strive to provide your patients with optimal oral care, your technical skill alone may not ensure success. You must also be able to communicate clearly to your patients the rationale for your treatment recommendations. Indeed, you may often find yourself in a position of trying to persuade patients to follow your advice. The intraoral camera can be of tremendous assistance in helping your patients understand and visualize conditions and the need for treatment, thus alleviating your "burden of proof" (Fig 3-7).

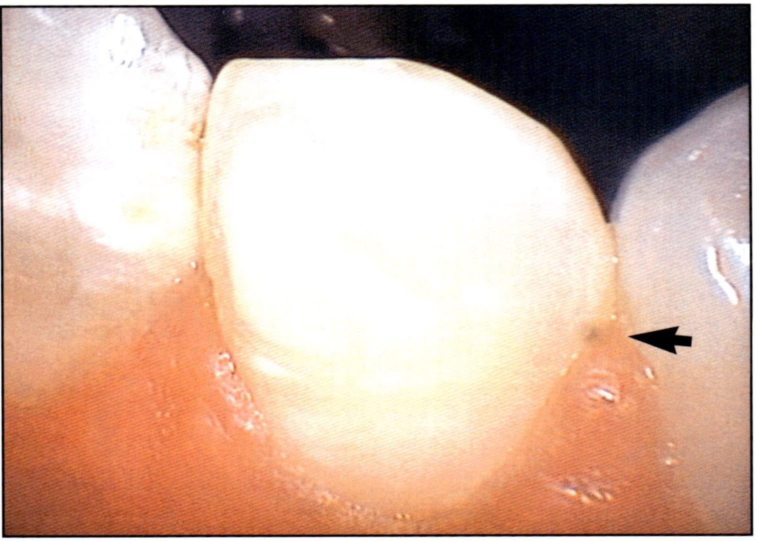

Fig 3-7 *Early signs of decay may not be visible to you or your patient without the aid of an intraoral camera.*

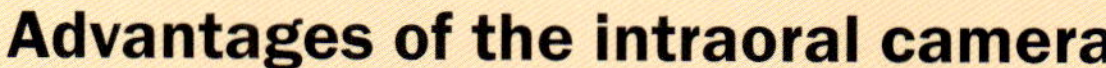

Advantages of the intraoral camera

1. Increased diagnostic assessment accuracy (10 to 40 times magnification)
   - Caries
   - Wear and fracture
   - Poor oral hygiene
   - Periodontal problems
2. Increased doctor-patient communication
3. Increased patient understanding
4. Increased trust in doctor
5. Increased patient role in treatment planning
6. Increased case acceptance rate
7. Improved documentation
   - Patient identification pictures for the chart
   - Insurance photos for increased third-party approval
8. Decreased consultation time
9. Higher staff morale
10. Increased patient referrals
11. Increased productivity due to decreased diagnostic time and increased patient acceptance
12. Perception of a state of the art "technologically advanced" practice
13. Documentation for malpractice or other legal situations

Intraoral Camera Technology

Intraoral cameras have been adapted for dentistry from medical endoscopic units, and many different types exist. The cameras are similar in size and shape to dental handpieces. Each of the available models has different optics and offers different advantages. Evaluate several before making a choice.

The specialized video intraoral cameras use solid-state imaging technology known as a charge coupled device (CCD). The target viewing area is focused onto the CCD, which consists of an array of picture elements, or "pixels." Each pixel responds to the light falling upon it. The image is therefore sampled by each pixel; the greater the number of pixels, the higher the sampling resolution.

Regardless of the sampling resolution, the major disadvantage of video cameras is that they must rely on the established video standards that have changed little over the last 40 years. Some of these analog standards include

NTSC, PAL, SECAM, and S-video. A true digital camera, while still using a CCD, is not restricted in quality by the conversion to an analog video signal.

For maximum utilization in dental applications, intraoral cameras must offer high-quality *resolution* and *color fidelity*. Resolution determines how much detail, such as fine fractures, the camera can capture. Color fidelity refers to the system's ability to accurately reproduce color. Faithful color reproduction, as well as the clear display of subtle color differences, can be critical to the detection of early caries, gingivitis, and precancerous lesions (Fig 3-8).

A high-quality lens is necessary for image excellence. Since the oral cavity is curved, a wide-angle lens with a corresponding curvature of field provides the best intraoral reproduction. This enables image quality to be maintained without constant refocusing.

Intraoral cameras may one day replace your intraoral mirrors.

Technological development in this field is continuing at a rapid pace. Cameras are becoming smaller while resolution and color fidelity are improving. Most cameras now have a built-in light source so that the target area is well illuminated. This direct light allows for the best color fidelity possible, since color is a reflection of light. Some camera systems, however, suggest using the ambient light within the operatory, combined with the overhead dental light source, rather than a light source built into the camera.

Initially, some camera systems provided a steady flow of air over the lens to prevent fogging, and hence a blurred image. Since a plastic sheath now covers most lens systems for sterilization purposes, fogging does not appear to be as much of a problem and a flow of air may be unnecessary. If there is fogging, use the air/water syringe to blow air over the lens.

Stand-alone video systems require a high-resolution color video monitor to view images captured by the intraoral camera. A color film printer will enable you to make hard copy images for the patient's record or insurance company (Fig 3-9). Additionally, an integrated computer will organize and store images in your patient's record for future reference. If your intraoral camera is integrated with a computer imaging system, you will be able to capture detailed images of the patient's mouth and modify them to illustrate proposed treatment options (Fig 3-10).

Intraoral cameras may one day replace your intraoral mirrors. You will be able to view the treatment area on a monitor, which will increase your view of the relative size of that area. These cameras can improve your results and your ease of accessibility, not to mention your posture!

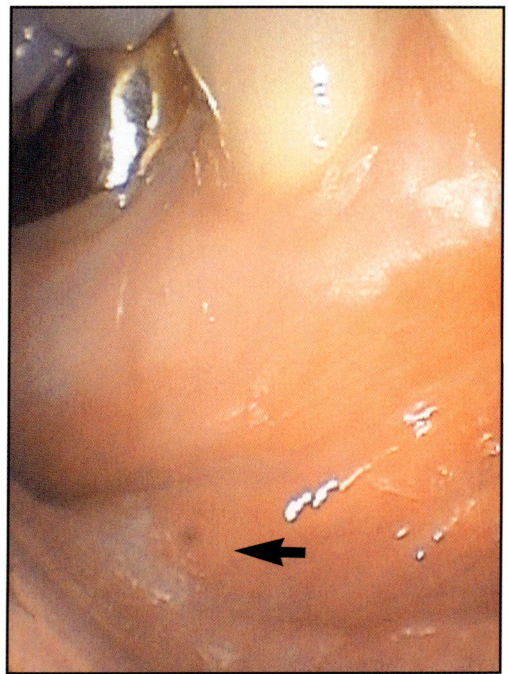

Fig 3-8 *Color fidelity is a must in detecting white lesions such as these.*

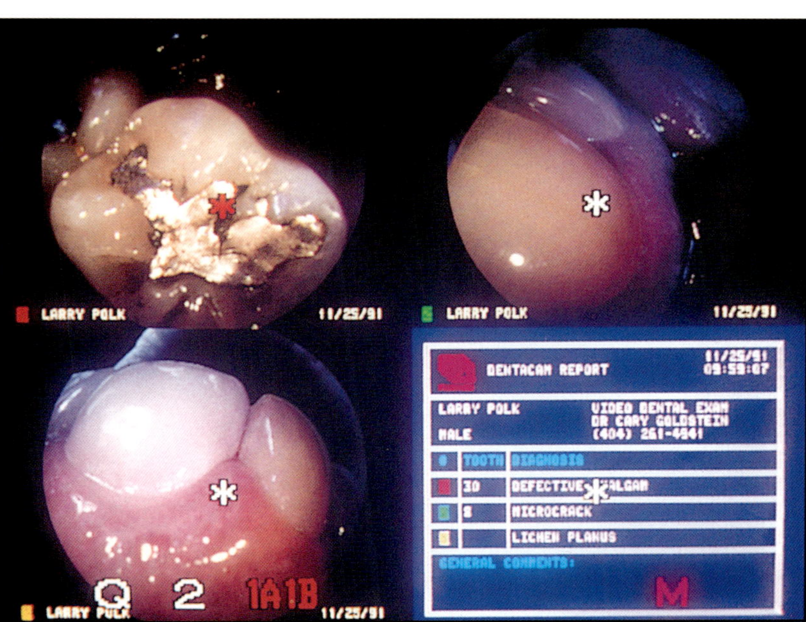

Fig 3-9 *Hard-copy prints are useful documentation for insurance companies.*

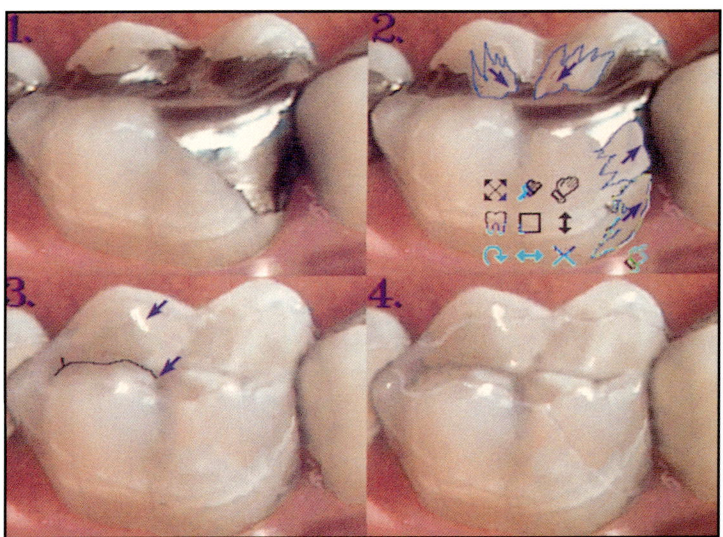

Fig 3-10 *Esthetic imaging is useful when patients do not understand your explanations of treatment options.*

Intraoral Video Network

An intraoral camera system can be located in an examination room or placed on a mobile cart, making it an easily accessible and fully portable diagnostic tool. Naturally, the smaller the camera system, the easier it will be to move between examination rooms. The use of one central imaging system placed in the office is becoming a popular option. This central unit allows you to have a monitor in any operatory and simply "plug in" the camera wherever needed. The printer, central processing unit (CPU), and storage device are left stationary in one operatory or even better, another more unobtrusive location (Fig 3-11).

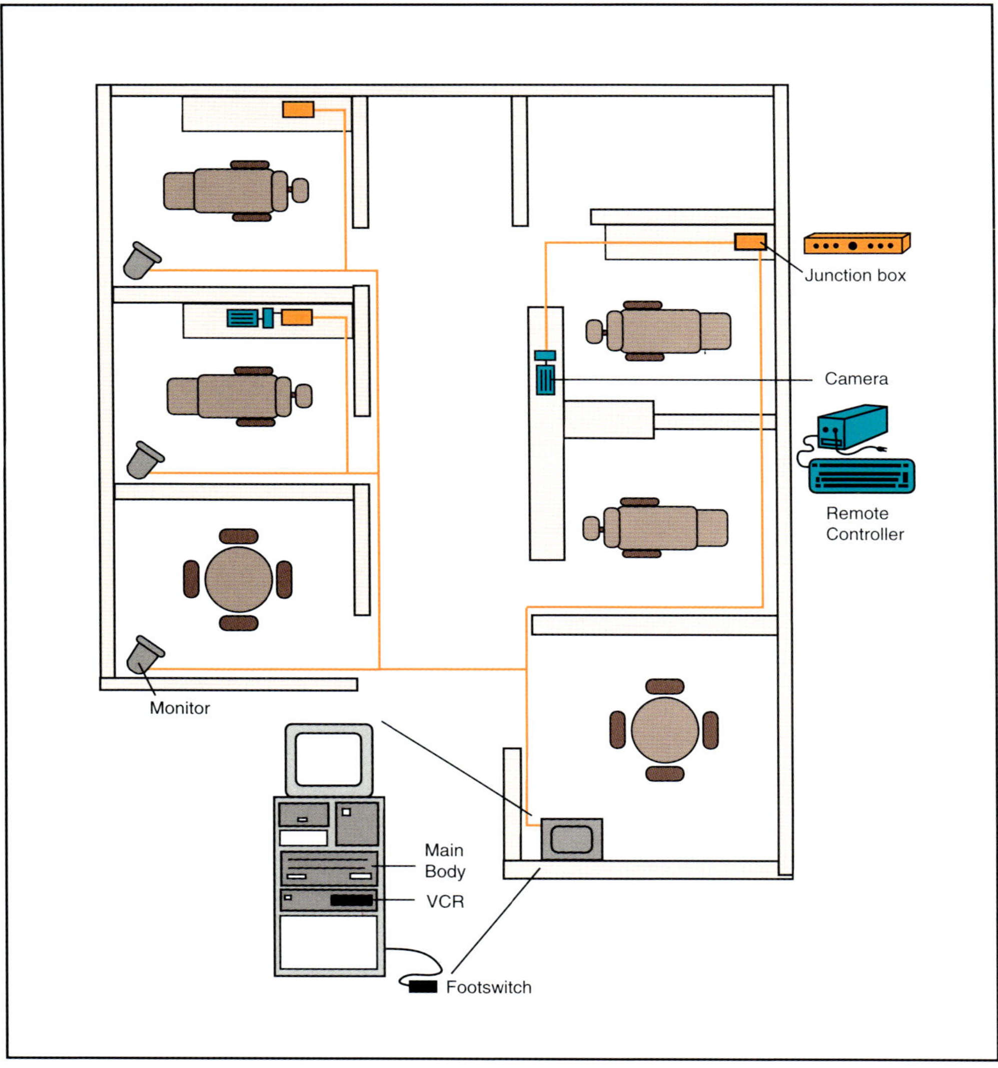

Fig 3-11 *This schematic drawing depicts a networked imaging system.*

The Print-Out

Whereas it is feasible to make an instant print of anything that is on the monitor, some companies include a reporting system allowing electronic communication with an insurance company so they can easily see the defect and reason for your treatment. A text report can accompany photos that can range from a part of a tooth to the entire arch, and even include a radiograph (Fig 3-12). Inclusion of a free text area allows you to describe your diagnosis of each tooth, with a space allocated for any additional comments you wish to make regarding your patient's status or treatment.

Unless you have adequate disk storage, you may wish to make three prints of the information–one for the patient, one for the insurance company, and one for your record. This type of report can be invaluable to the patient who has been in an accident and may have a legal situation. There is no better documentation of the extent of trauma (particularly microcracks) to the tooth. In the event your patient hires an attorney or uses the print-out as documentation for the insurance company, you will be providing visual information that can make settlement of the patient's claim much easier.

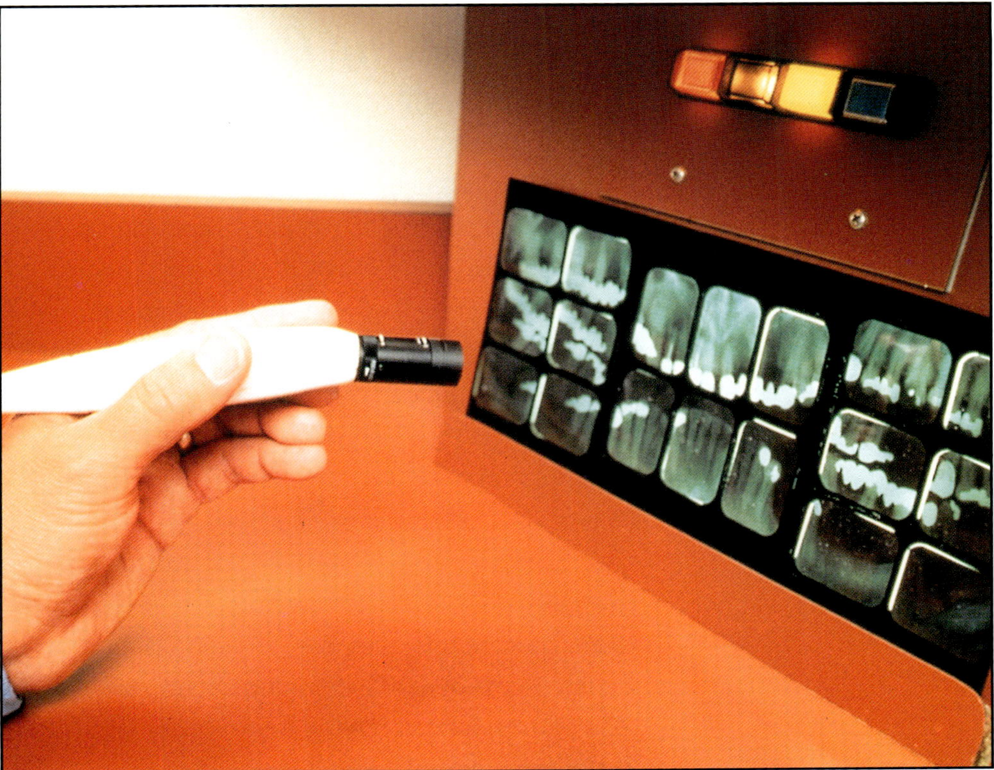

Fig 3-12 Your intraoral system can digitize radiographs for instant hard copies or for use in electronic claims filing.

Requirements for an intraoral video camera system

1. Camera and sterile sleeves
2. Light source
3. SVGA (high-resolution) monitor

Extra items you may want

1. Computer and software
2. Large screen monitor
3. VCR
4. Digital printer (color or b/w)
5. Video printer
6. LCD glasses for the patient
7. Extraoral camera
8. Scanner for slides and radiographs
9. Other dental software (eg, practice management system)
10. CD-ROM drive
11. Other computer-based peripherals

Incorporating the Intraoral Camera into Your Practice

A video tour of the mouth provides a "more comprehensive and educational examination process."[1] You can expect your patients to ask more questions, become more involved in the diagnostic process, and have a better understanding and acceptance of your treatment goals.

Ideally, your patient should view the exam on the monitor with you. Unfortunately, unless the monitor is strategically positioned, this may prove difficult. Products that incorporate small LCD (liquid crystal display) panels in an "eyeglass" apparatus make patient viewing easy without interfering with your field of vision (Fig 3-13a). Alternatively, place a monitor in your ceiling (3-13b).

To enhance your productivity, the intraoral video exam may be delegated to an assistant or hygienist who has sufficient expertise in the use of the equipment. Be sure this person is someone who:

1. Has excellent verbal communication skills
2. Is enthusiastic about the intraoral camera
3. Has considerable dental experience
4. Receives personalized training from you on what you expect them to accomplish

While you are treating a patient, your assistant or a hygienist can be working with a different patient. The auxiliary can review a patient's intraoral condition, discuss possible treatment options, assist with any questions the patient may have, and help to prepare for and focus on his or her diagnostic consultation with you. Once you enter the treatment room, the patient will be informed of the problem areas and educated about his or her needed treatment. You will need only to review and verify the diagnosis and suggested treatment.

The intraoral camera, which is relatively simple to use, is held much like an explorer or a handpiece, and is passed slowly over the teeth and tissue. Make sure the teeth are dry so that the defects are revealed accurately. The enlarged tooth and tissue images on the monitor help facilitate detection of cracks, leaking margins, or other areas of pathology. Again, having your patient view these defects as you do can be of enormous help in motivating the patient to seek the proper treatment.

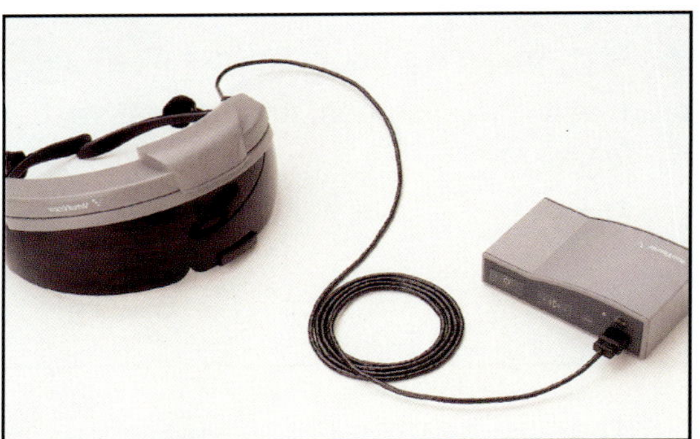

Fig 3-13a *Video monitors incorporated into an "eyeglass" apparatus make viewing by your patient easy without restricting operator view.*

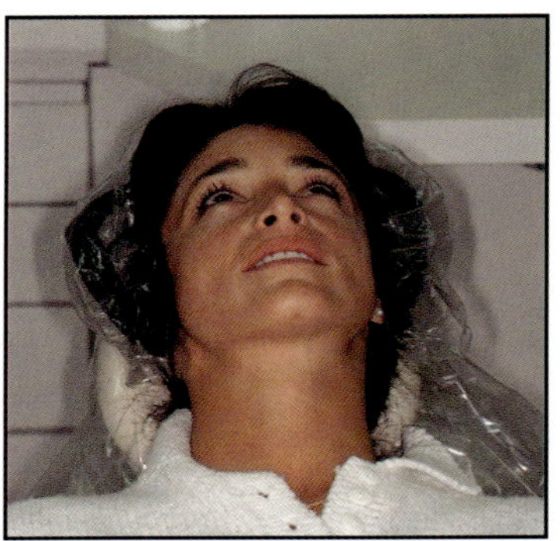

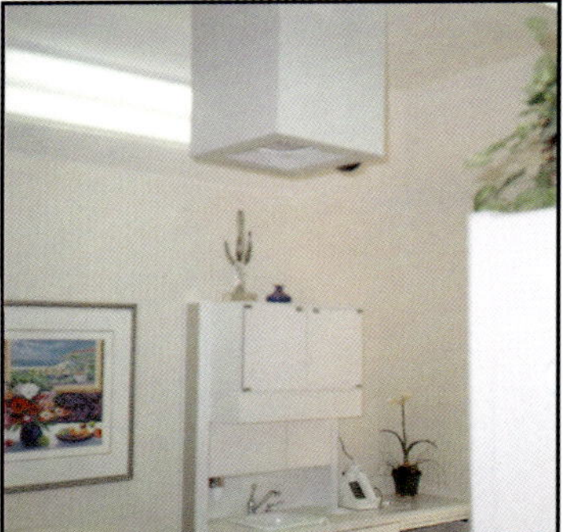

Fig 3-13b *Incorporating a monitor in your ceiling makes it easy for your patient to view the video exam, and it can also act as a patient entertainment system.*

Practice Enhancement

Research has shown that practices using the intraoral video camera may have up to twice the referral rate of practices that do not use it.[2] The probable explanation is that patients enthusiastically relate their intraoral imaging experience to others and inspire them to seek out this technology for their own dental care. In fact, in time, patients may come to view the lack of use of this technology as inferior and irresponsible dentistry.

A recent survey of dentists using intraoral cameras gave five reasons for its success:[3]

1. Increases case acceptance
2. Increases practice productivity
3. Increases new patients and referrals
4. Increases staff motivation and retention
5. Decreases time needed for diagnostic consultation

Intraoral systems can be leased or purchased. Since the average U.S. dental practice will produce approximately $400 per new patient and the intraoral camera can increase that figure between 200% and 400%, it is no wonder that these cameras have become so popular.[2]

The following are three possible methods for incorporating the intraoral camera into your practice:

1. The intraoral video exam can be included in your normal examination fee.
2. A small fee can be added to your regular exam fee when the intraoral camera is used.
3. A separate intraoral exam fee can be charged and the fee could be applied to any dental treatment.

Used correctly, the intraoral camera will enhance your practice. As Levin suggests, use the camera with every patient—make it a habit. Never talk about an oral condition without having a picture of it on the screen. An intraoral system is an invaluable investment in your practice![4]

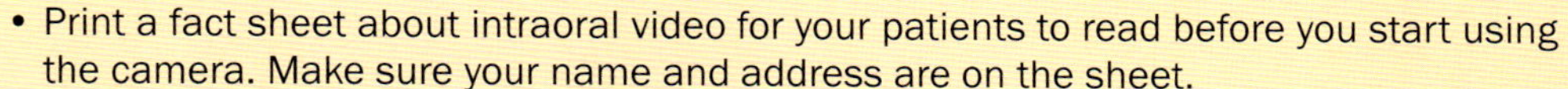

Practice enhancement tips for the intraoral camera

- Print a fact sheet about intraoral video for your patients to read before you start using the camera. Make sure your name and address are on the sheet.
- Print before-and-after treatment pictures for your patients; they may show these pictures to their friends, family, and coworkers. (Your name, phone number and address should be on the prints.)
- Prepare a catalogue of before-and-after images of completed patient treatments so that patients may review the various treatments that you have provided, such as bleaching, cosmetic contouring, and laminates. (If full face images are used, be sure to receive written permission from your patient.)
- Send hard-copy intraoral images to the insurance company to document the need for treatment when radiographic images alone may be insufficient.
- Educate your staff, including nonclinical personnel, on how the camera works and its advantages. Remember, your front-office staff has the initial contact with patients.
- Spotlight this new technology in a letter to your patients, your newsletter, and in handouts in the reception area.

Considerations in buying an intraoral camera

1. Resolution—the detail of the on-screen image (the higher the number of pixels and horizontal lines, the better the resolution)
2. Color fidelity—accuracy of color reproduction
3. Lack of distortion
4. Camera type—CCD (charge coupled device). The scene to be viewed is focused onto the CCD, which consists of an array of picture elements (pixels), each of which responds to the light falling upon it. The image is sampled by each pixel; the greater the number of pixels, the higher the sampling resolution.
5. Digital images
   - Direct
   - Indirect (uses a mirror and produces a reversed image)
6. Illumination
   - Ambient
   - Direct
7. Size of the camera head
   - Smaller is better
   - Must give access to difficult-to-see areas
8. Sterility
   - Heat sterilized, cold sterilized, or a plastic sleeve?
9. Portability
   - Ease; one plug; few wires
   - Increased use results in faster return on investment
   - Central unit option with movable camera
10. Defog capability
    - Air stream
    - Defog liquid
    - Permanent coating on the lens

References

1. Levin RP. Building your practice with an intraoral video camera. Compendium 1990;11:52.
2. Lackey AD. Intra-oral video photography: questions and answers. J Calif Dent Assoc 1991;19(3):29–30.
3. Healthcare Advancements; 1989 Survey. The intraoral video camera explained.
4. Levin RP. Selling More Dentistry with the Intraoral Camera. Baltimore: The Levin Group, 1993.

Further Reading

Goldstein RE, Miller MC. High technology in esthetic dentistry. Curr Opin Cosmet Dent 1993:5–11.

Markowitz SS. Video imaging machines and intraoral cameras. Alpha Omegan 1991;84:25–26.

Bonner P. Intraoral video camera systems. Dentistry Today 1992;11:72–75.

Video and audio tapes

Christensen G. Effective Use of Intraoral Video (#V4770). Practical Clinical Courses, Provo, Utah.

Knall P. 52 Applications of the Intraoral Video. Citadel Dentistry, Scottsdale, Arizona.

Electronic *Imaging* Technology

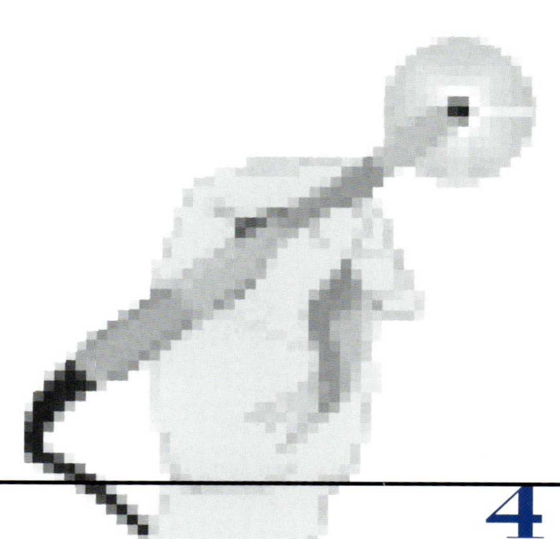

4

Intraoral systems, adapted from endoscopes used in medicine, provide the missing link in the communications chain between dentists and patients.

Images are a significant, even critical, component in the delivery of health care. Medical professionals rely on advanced imaging technologies such as computed tomography (CT) and magnetic resonance imaging (MRI) to obtain and record care-related information. And while radiographic and photographic images have been a mainstay in dentistry, the introduction of the intraoral camera can be credited as the most significant catalyst for advancing imaging awareness. Intraoral systems, adapted from endoscopes used in medicine, provide the missing link in the communications chain between dentists and patients (Figs 4-1 and 4-2).

Essentially, intraoral cameras are used in place of traditional hand mirrors. Designed specifically for use in the oral cavity, most intraoral cameras have a slender lens and lighting system and produce a standard video signal, which is relayed to a computer and digitized for viewing on a monitor. These "live" intraoral images are magnified on the screen to become an effective diagnostic tool. Typical video-based intraoral systems use video printers to freeze a frame of video for diagnosis and produce full-color photographic quality prints to permanently record an image.

As with any advanced technology, imaging is not without its own unique shortcomings. There are many sources for images used in dentistry. A wide variety of images are acquired through many different mechanisms and stored on different media. Hard-copy images from radiographs, intraoral prints, and photographic slides are usually stored separately from the patient record in carousels, trays, and sleeve and file folders. This visual information is not organized in a unified, seamless manner, nor is it well integrated with other information in the patient record. Collecting all visual documentation for even a single episode of care is frequently cumbersome.

Advances in computer technology are providing innovative solutions for the specific needs of dentistry. Today, with the proliferation of imaging technologies, increasing numbers of practitioners recognize the need for a comprehensive system to manage the vast numbers of images they produce, store, and access during the diagnostic, treatment planning, and therapeutic phases of patient care. Sophisticated image management is becoming a requirement to assist dental professionals in their decision-making processes.

The evolution of the personal computer has spawned a revolution in the development of new opportunities in dentistry. Computer-based systems first appeared as proprietary stand-alone solutions designed to address specific segments, such as practice management, periodontal charting, cosmetic imaging, radiology, and, to some degree, intraoral video. These systems, usually self-contained, were installed on their own carts with their own processors, and each took up a significant amount of space. Further, these stand-alone systems did not share data, and therefore redundant information such as name and medical record number had to be separately entered into each system. Although each of these products addressed a unique requirement, combining their functions into a single multipurpose platform—the clinical workstation—is the current goal.

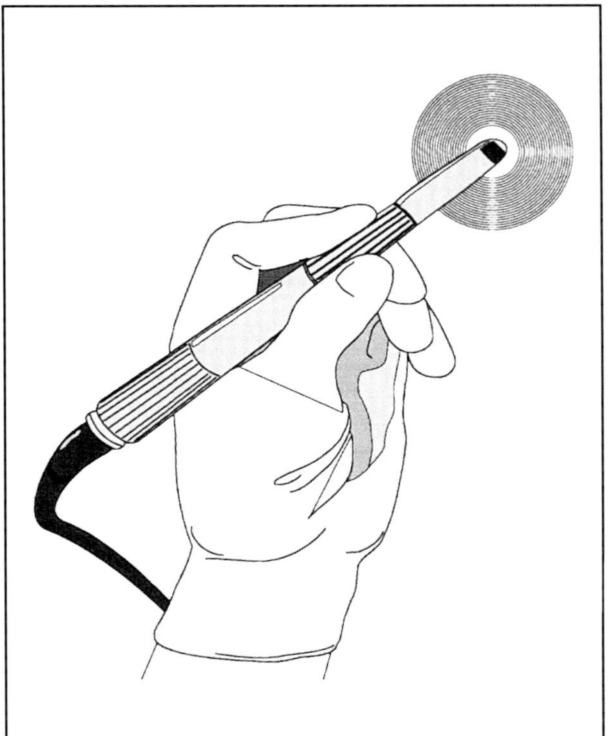

Fig 4-1 Essentially, intraoral cameras are used in place of traditional hand mirrors.

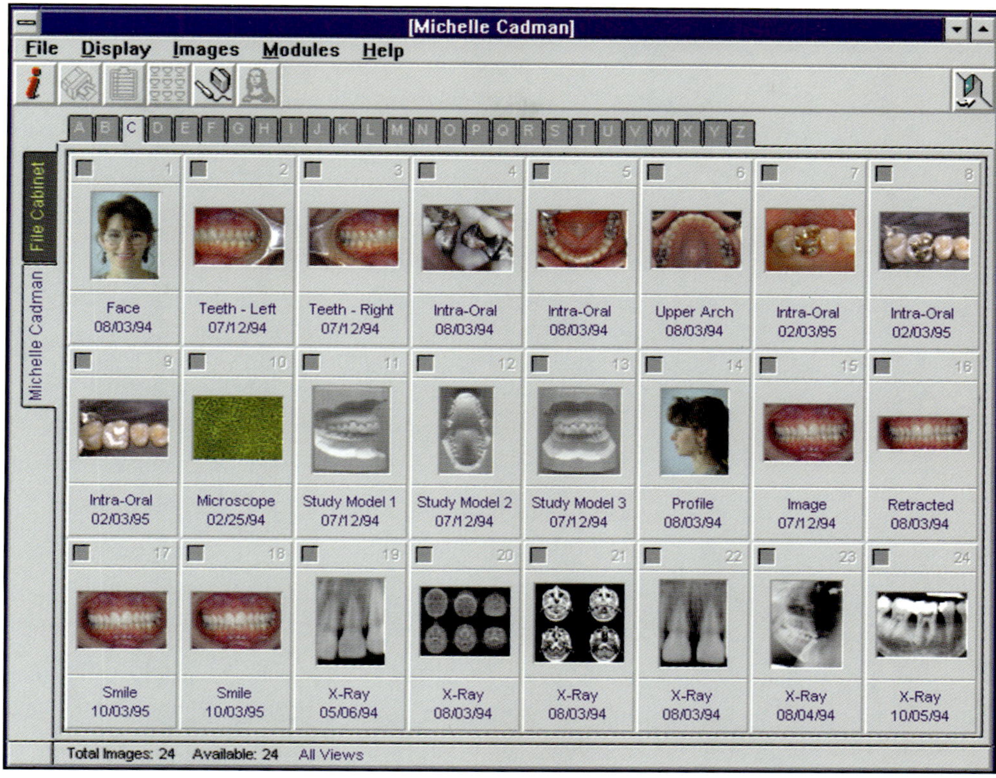

Fig 4-2 Example of an image database. Visual media should always be used for documentation and reference in treatment planning.

System Integration

The workstation provides a computer hardware platform where dentists and auxiliaries can input and review clinical data and prepare treatment plans in many locations, including chairside. With a complete patient record available from one workstation (rather than from multiple independent systems found in different locations throughout the office), dental providers can use the computer's power in their decision-making and treatment process. Images are an integral component of the decision process. According to *The Computer Based Oral Health Record,*[1] a clinical workstation should include an image-management software module for digital radiographs and intraoral and extraoral color photographs. Visual media should always be used for documentation and reference in treatment planning.

Imaging Hardware

Personal computer companies are producing systems to meet the demands of the most advanced dental imaging applications. PCs are based on a wide variety of central processing unit (CPU) architectures designed by many manufacturers such as Intel, Motorola, and others. Performance can range from adequate to spectacular, but they are all designed to do three things: accept data (from the user and installed devices); store data to be accessed at a later date; and provide access to the stored data for modeling and analysis.

As the power of desktop computers has increased, the majority of the PC market has divided into two main architectures. The first is based on a family of computer processor chips from Intel Corporation. The list of system manufacturers utilizing the Intel chips includes corporate giants such as IBM, Compaq, Hewlett Packard, as well as many "clone" or IBM-compatible suppliers. The other architecture is Apple Computer whose Macintosh line is based on a CPU from Motorola. There are pros and cons for implementing either architecture, but this chapter is not intended to address this debate. With either CPU design, there are some common safeguards to look for and pitfalls to avoid.

Imaging imposes heavy demands on a system's resources, both memory and storage. It is common for today's operating systems (OS), with their graphical user interfaces (GUI), to require a minimum of 16 Mb of system memory (RAM—random access memory), with 32 Mb recommended. While this is significant, it should be noted that an image file can easily occupy 1 Mb or more of hard-drive space. When evaluating computer systems for imaging, expandability is probably your most important consideration. Your computer needs will change as your understanding and use of imaging grows. Make sure your system vendor plans for future expandability and configures a system that can grow with you. Constant technology development makes obsolescence a major concern. This can be combated with advance planning that adheres to the philosophy of industry standards and upgrading rather than replacing system components.

Memory

A computer requires memory, both in the form of system RAM and hard-drive capacity, to provide a "work space" for the OS and the application software to manipulate data. The relative cost of memory is decreasing to allow for a sufficient amount of system memory (RAM) to optimize a system's performance. Memory modules, used in nearly every PC system, are small circuit boards that bundle memory chips together and plug into special sockets on your computer's system board. Adding more memory to a system is relatively straightforward, provided there are available memory module sockets. If not, the only way to increase your available RAM is to remove some of the existing memory modules and replace them with higher capacity modules, provided your system supports them. Keep in mind that it is more cost-effective to configure your system with room for RAM expansion.

Hard drives are not as fast in relation to a system's RAM, but provide a relatively quick and cost-effective form of on-line storage. Installing a high-capacity hard drive will ensure that your application programs and data files are accessible in a reasonable time frame. As mentioned before, image files can be large, and therefore an imaging system should be configured with a high-capacity hard drive to ensure efficient file storage and access. If there were no hard drive or other mass storage device available, it would be physically impossible, with current limitations of PC architecture, for an imaging system to be configured with enough RAM to hold everything (OS, programs, and data files) in memory at one time.

Hard disk drives are the most mechanical component of any computer system, and therefore the most susceptible to failure. Regular backup of critical data from the hard disk is prudent. As hard-disk space becomes limited due to the capability of on-line storage, it may become necessary to archive older data. Two devices are available for this type of off-line storage, tape backup and WORM (write once, read many) laser disk drives. Tape backup systems are inexpensive but sometimes unreliable; WORM drives produce CD-size laser disks and are extremely reliable.

Memory-related questions to ask when purchasing imaging hardware

1. How much RAM (random access memory) is installed in the system?
2. Can I add additional RAM? If so, how much?
3. Can I keep the existing RAM and simply add additional chips to increase the memory? If not, what is involved?
4. What size is the hard drive (MB or GB)? Is it enough?
5. Can I easily upgrade the hard drive to a higher capacity in the future?
6. Can I add a tape backup or WORM drive?

Graphics Subsystem

The next area to consider in your imaging system is the computer's display. Sometimes called the graphics subsystem, the display is composed of two components, the display monitor and the display adapter. The display components should be carefully matched to achieve the best overall picture quality for viewing images. To effectively view the full-color images acquired with an imaging system, your graphics subsystem should be capable of 15-bit color display, at a minimum (Fig 4-3a to e). Most display monitors are analog, meaning they can display virtually an unlimited number of colors, **so it is important to remember that it is the *display adapter*, and not the monitor, that determines the number of colors your system can present for viewing.**

If your imaging system uses a display adapter that is not capable of a minimum of least 15-bit color (32,768 simultaneous colors), your imaging application will suffer by having to "translate" or map the image colors to match the available display colors. This procedure is known as palette matching and is generally accompanied by a color-reduction process called *dithering,* in which a pattern of available colors is used to simulate others. The result is an image that is not accurately represented on your monitor. Fortunately, high-end graphics adapters are no longer a luxury. High-quality, high-performance display adapters are available for the same price as their low-color peers were a few short years ago, so it is worthwhile to include one in your imaging system.

When selecting a monitor, the main considerations are screen size (measured diagonally), dot pitch, and video refresh rate. Large screen monitors are becoming more affordable, but before choosing the latest 21-inch model, consider the space limitations of your operatory.

The number of colors an adapter can display at different pixel depths

Bits per pixel	Available colors
4	16
8	256
15	32,768
16	65,536
24	16,777,216

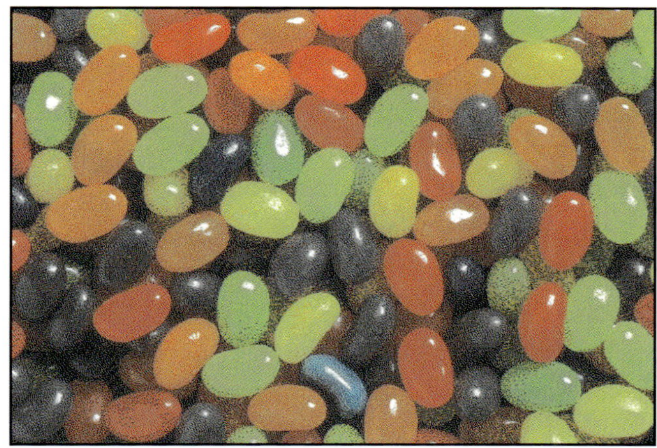

Fig 4-3a *Four-bit color image contains only 16 dithered colors. Dithering is a color-reduction process in which a pattern of available colors is used to simulate other colors.*

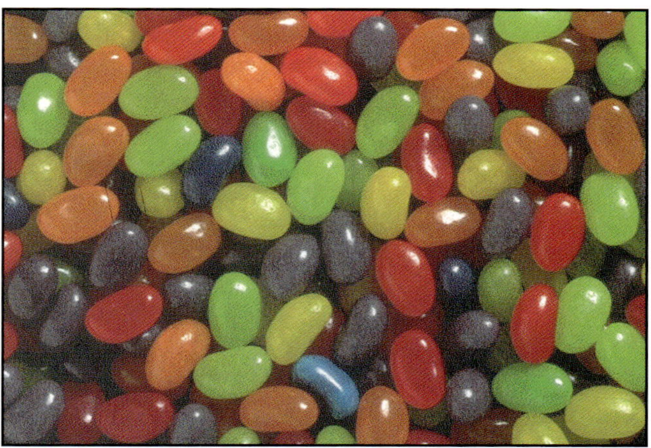

Fig 4-3b *Eight-bit color image contains 256 dithered colors.*

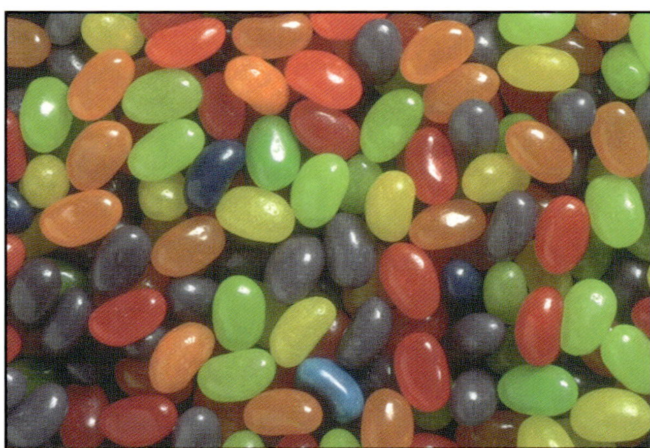

Fig 4-3c *Fifteen-bit color image contains 32,768 dithered colors.*

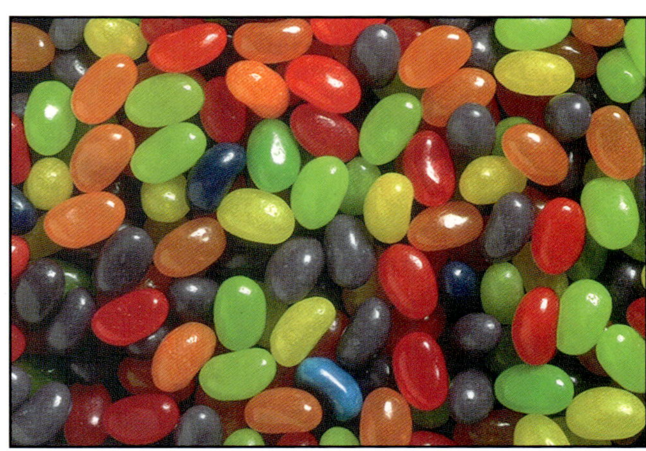

Fig 4-3d *Sixteen-bit color image contains 65,536 dithered colors.*

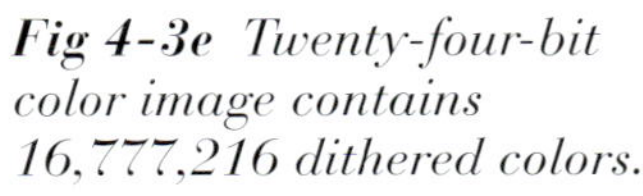

Fig 4-3e *Twenty-four-bit color image contains 16,777,216 dithered colors.*

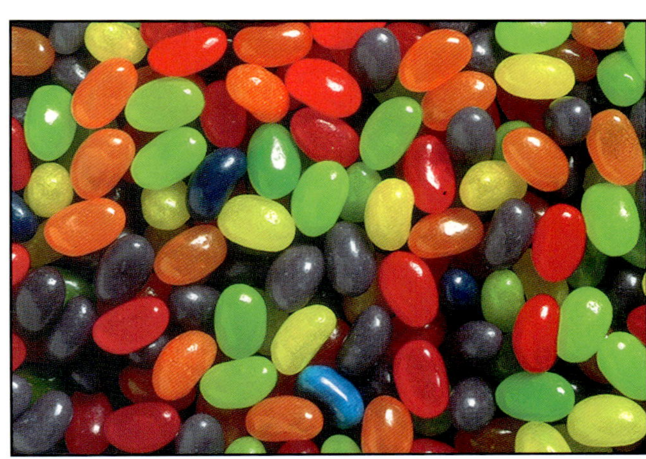

The dot pitch specification of the a monitor refers to the space, in millimeters (mm), separating the color-producing pixels on the screen. Individual pixels produce red, green, and blue colors, and when displayed in combination, they approximate virtually every color available. If the space between these pixels is too great, the image will not appear focused: the smaller the dot pitch, the sharper an image will appear. While a 0.28-mm dot pitch can be sufficient, models with a 0.26-mm dot pitch or less are affordable. **Look for the smallest dot pitch to ensure a quality image on screen** (Fig 4-4).

Another technical area to consider for the monitor is the video refresh rate, because a correct match with your display adapter is most critical. While most of today's monitors can synchronize to a wide range of frequencies (sometimes called MultiSync), they generally work best at a specific video refresh rate. The default frequency of a typical display adapter is 60 Hz, but it is advisable to look for a higher frequency combination to minimize the visible flicker that the graphics subsystem can create. **Rather than burying yourself in technical specifications, simply observe the available graphics subsystem options and buy the monitor/display adapter combination that looks best to you.**

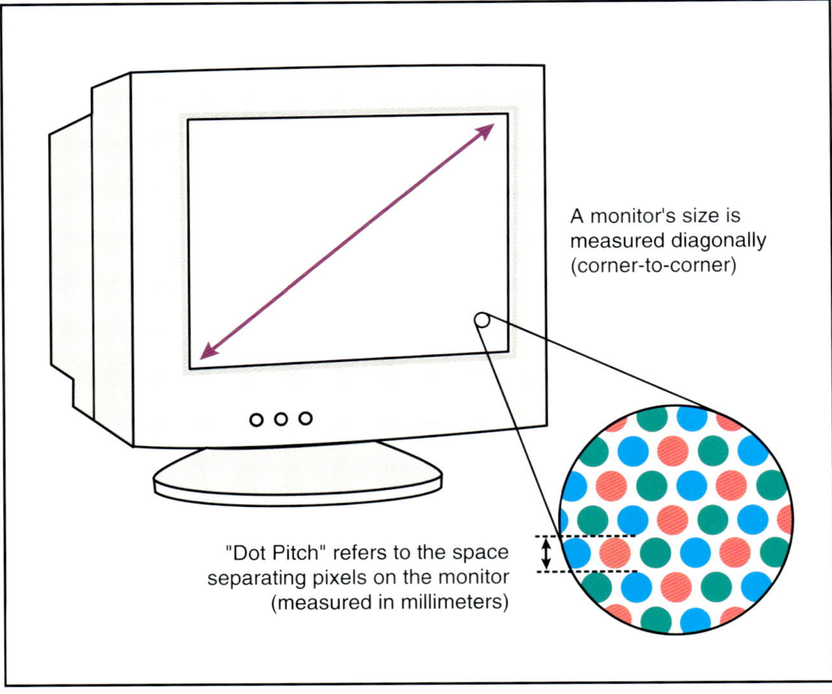

Fig 4-4 *A monitor's size is measured diagonally. Choose a monitor with a large enough screen size and the lowest dot pitch, which is the space separating color-producing pixels.*

Video Framegrabber

Computerization has created a new method of storing information—digitally. "Digitization" organizes data in a complex combination of ones and zeros to represent all data, including images. One of the most difficult goals to achieve when connecting a video source, such as an intraoral camera, to a computer, is converting an analog video signal into a digital image in real-time.

Analog video has existed in its present form since the advent of television. While innovations, such as color, have been introduced over the years, the basic video standard remains unchanged. If you were to connect a television from the 1950s to a high-tech intraoral camera today, you would be able to see a picture, albeit in black and white. Because the standards for video were set decades ago, video technology that adheres to these standards must be backwards compatible. These analog video standards use a process called interlacing. This means that the monitor scans odd and even lines on separate passes. This reduces screen motion flutter. Because digital images typically are used in still frame and do not require interlacing, the monitor should be "non-interlaced" to produce a crisp image.

In converting a video signal into a digital format, a specialized adapter called a *framegrabber* is used. Framegrabbers were initially expensive, but growing market awareness and competition have helped to drive down the price. But be aware that this is still a very specialized product, and the quality of your digitized image can vary greatly. Not every framegrabber will work with every display adapter. Usually it is the video refresh rate that restricts a framegrabber and a display adapter from working together. This is not a hardware deficiency on the part of the framegrabber, but a design implementation, on the part of the display adapter manufacturer, to try to optimize the performance of the product.

In converting a video signal into a digital format, a specialized adapter called a framegrabber *is used.*

PC architecture imposes many limitations on hardware engineers. At times, the design of a high-performance peripheral sacrifices some industry standards. Inevitably you will be faced with incompatible hardware issues. Your imaging software vendor or consultant can provide recommendations for the framegrabber product that best suits your system. Although framegrabbers digitize analog video and theoretically work with any intraoral camera that produces an industry standard video signal, knowledgeable selection is paramount.

Specialized Imaging Equipment

The intraoral camera is only one of several devices that captures images. Still-photography cameras (35 mm) and radiographic equipment have been used for years in dentistry for treatment planning, record documentation, history documentation, case presentation, diagnosis, identification, and analysis. Converting these images for use and storage in a computer-based system, however, requires specialized equipment.

Photo CD. Kodak has designed one solution for converting existing still photos into a digital format called Photo CD whereby a photo processor scans stills, negatives, or slides and stores the images on a compact disk (CD). The Photo CD format can store up to 100 images that can be accessed by a compatible CD-ROM drive. Unless you have your own in-house film-processing facility, Photo CDs will require that you send your film out for development. In the same time it takes to develop your pictures, a Photo CD developer will digitize and store your images on a disk. This offers a reasonably cost-effective method of digitizing your pictures while you continue to use the same photographic procedure as always. Once your photographs are digitized on the CD, you can view them with your (Photo CD–compatible) imaging application software.

In the same time it takes to develop your pictures, a Photo CD developer will digitize and store your images on a disk.

If you decide to use Photo CDs in your practice, the most important issues to consider when purchasing a Photo CD–compliant CD-ROM drive are *data access time* and *multi-session photo CD support*. CD-ROM drives range in price and quality, so look for a drive that offers the best performance within your budget. Many drives specify that they support Photo CD, but they may support only single sessions. Even if a Photo CD can store up to 100 images, it should not mean that you have to put them on the CD all at once. You may have only a handful that you need digitized at any particular time. Any images you choose to put on the disk later will be saved in additional "sessions." If your CD-ROM drive does not support multi-session Photo CDs, you will not be able to access the images you stored in the previous sessions.

Digital Radiography Equipment. Many companies are in conflict over other direct digital imaging solutions, particularly dental radiographic equipment. Some manufacturers are using a "wired" sensor, which, when bombarded with X-rays, is directly stimulated to produce an image through a proprietary interface board installed in your computer. Others use X-ray sensitive plates that can be scanned with proprietary laser readers, linked to a computer, to produce an image. Direct digital X-ray technology appears to be gaining favor in the market. The manufacturers claim a reduction in radiation exposure time (from 70% to 90%) vs the conventional. While this is better for the patient, traditional radiographic equipment is still required for total diagnostic integrity.

Scanners. Large format radiographs, such as panoramics and cephalometrics, are, because of their size, a challenge for any direct digital format. There has been some progress toward a direct digital solution for these formats, but at this point the costs are too prohibitive. Computer scanners are one solution for digitizing larger X-ray films. Scanners come in a number of configurations, with the "flatbed" scanner as the most common style. Not unlike the top portion of a photocopier machine, a flatbed scanner requires you to align your image on the glass surface. Through the computer interface, you control the quality, size, and resolution of the scanned image. Unfortunately, scanners are not designed for the novice user. They are constantly in need of alignment, and only an experienced operator will achieve consistently satisfactory results. Also, the quality of a scanner can vary greatly, with the associated costs ranging from under $1,000 to tens of thousands of dollars.

Once you have found a scanner that meets your needs and falls within your price range, be sure that it supports a standard software interface known as *TWAIN*. TWAIN has emerged as the most prominent software interface for scanners, so purchasing a TWAIN-compliant device will ensure that your scanner can be used by any software application that also supports TWAIN.

While digital media are convenient for both acquisition and storage, the fact that images are digitized does not necessarily mean that they will be any more organized than before.

Digital-image acquisition devices are constantly evolving. There are now digital alternatives to your 35-mm camera and maybe even your intraoral camera. The common element in all of the emerging digital image acquisition technologies is the computer, so it is important that digital solutions are flexible enough to co-exist with other imaging solutions. Proprietary computer interfaces are often required, especially with new technologies, so be sure that any specialized product you choose will not conflict with your existing system.

It is important to note that while digital media are convenient for both acquisition and storage, the fact that images are digitized does not necessarily mean that they will be any more organized than before. You will still need the power of an image-management software application to compile your images into a concise catalogue to be effectively used in your practice.

Additional System Components

There are additional components that you will need to consider to effectively implement a complete imaging system in your practice. Previously we discussed the use of a graphical user interface (GUI), generally a part of the operating system (OS) installed on your system. A GUI is considered to be more "user-friendly" than a command-line, or function key, alternative. It uses a pointing device to help navigate around the screen and allows access to the functions of the operating system and software applications.

Pointing Devices. A "mouse" is the most common pointing device used with PCs. Other types of pointing devices include graphics tablets, track balls, light pens, and touch screens. While they can vary greatly in their form and function, all pointing devices ultimately accomplish the same basic task of providing a mechanism to "point and click" at the commands visible on the screen. When choosing a pointing device, make sure it is comfortable in your hand and allows you a reasonable amount of flexibility in order to take advantage of the graphical capabilities of your imaging application.

Communication Considerations. Another hardware component to consider is a modem. Short for "modulate/demodulate," a modem provides a digital link to the outside world via standard telephone lines. A modem is recommended for two reasons: vendor technical support staff can communicate with your system to correct many problems remotely; and with the appropriate software, information, such as images, can be transmitted electronically to laboratories and colleagues.

As with every aspect of the computer industry, modem technology is not immune to advancement. It is recommended that your modem performs at the highest industry-standard data-transfer rate available (measured in bits per second, and sometimes referred to as baud rate), while still maintaining backward compatibility with the older standards. Many new modems use a digital signal processor (DSP) chip and advanced telephony technology. DSP-based modems offer a distinct advantage over standard modems in that they are software upgradable. Initially they cost more than traditional modems but, as the communication standards improve, you can upgrade your DSP modem to keep pace with the advancements.

Internet Access. With the introduction of the World Wide Web, the internet has added a graphical user interface to allow internet access for the general population. No longer is it necessary to suffer the long learning process of the previous command-line interface. The Web enables users to access vast amounts of information as well as directly communicate with others who have similar needs or interests. In health-care delivery, the Web provides for the transmission and reception of both data and images for consulting purposes at a relatively low cost because it eliminates both long-distance and postal charges.

The key to the use of the Web is the selection of the internet service provider (ISP). The ISP can be compared to your local telephone company, and in some cases may be just that, as more local phone companies are offering internet access. The performance of your internet access is related to the speed of your access device. Access devices can be a modem, an ISDN (integrated services digital network) interface, or even cable television.

Currently, most ISDNs provide for modem speeds of 28.8 KBPS (kilobits per second), and some are beginning to offer up to 56 KBPS reception capability. However, modems seem to be reaching the upper speed limits that can be supported by current band-width technology. ISDN offers speeds of 128 KBPS but requires sophisticated set-up parameters that must be coordinated with the local phone company and the ISP. This technology also seems to be close to its maximum speed limitations. The newest internet access is through cable, or fiber optics. This system is now being tested in various areas around the U.S. and is providing access speeds of 200 KBPS with future accelerated speeds anticipated.

Networking

A computer network provides the framework, or backbone, for achieving complete practice information integration, enabling information and images to be accessible throughout the office and even from remote locations such as the dentist's home. Local area networks (LANs) are available in many forms. The most basic is generally referred to as a peer-to-peer network. As the name implies, all computers in a peer-to-peer network are equal. Each can allow the others access to its resources, including programs, files, and printers. However, peer-to-peer networks suffer from their inability to completely protect data from unauthorized access or corruption. It takes a much higher level of sophistication to provide a secured network. This generally means dedicating a computer to act as a "server" for the system to manage the network. When a workstation requests services from the server, the request will be authorized and processed only if the security requirements of the system have been met (Fig 4-5).

As your practice, and subsequently your system, grows, and more computers are connected, it may become necessary to look at a server-based solution to effectively address your network requirements. For the larger dental practice or clinic environment, it may be wise to consider a powerful UNIX-based LAN backbone server. These systems provide scaleable architectures, redundancy, and massive data storage capabilities.

Realistically, every practice will have its own unique scenario and you may wish to consult a qualified networking professional to help make an educated decision. Remember, with the right network interface adapters (NICs) and appropriate wiring configuration, a simple system can easily grow and adapt as your needs change.

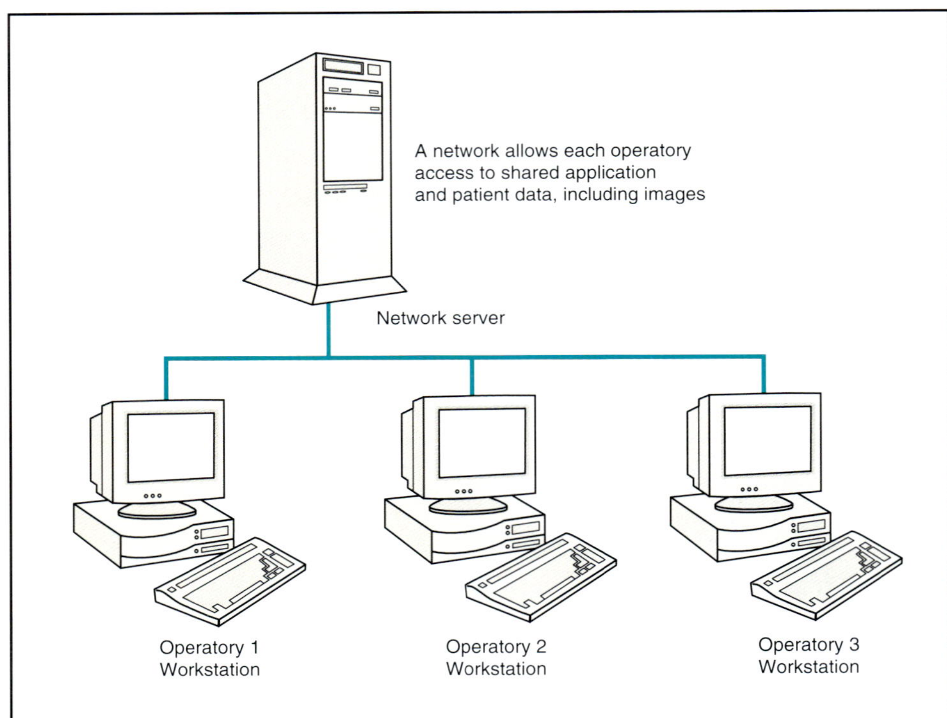

Fig 4-5 *A server is the "manager" of the network. Each workstation requests services from the server.*

An Open Upgrade Pathway

The essential issue with any imaging solution is an open upgrade pathway to allow your system to grow with you. The first step into the world of imaging technology should not be taken lightly, but at the same time you should not be afraid to take that step. The right solutions will not only enhance your practice, but also provide you with additional tools that will assist you in making appropriate, even exceptional, clinical decisions.

Reference

1. Eisner J, Chasteen JE, Schleyer T, et al. The Computer-Based Oral Health Record. The AADS Consortium for Clinical Information Systems, 1993.

Software Overview

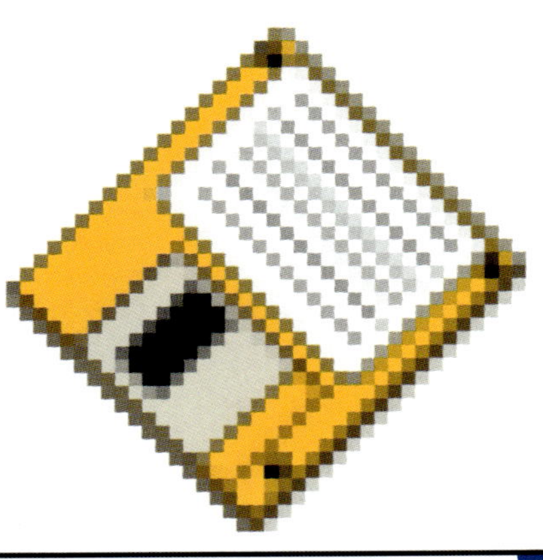

5

Wayne Rees

Computer advancements are propelling us into the interactive age. Dental office automation used to mean a computerized business software application running on a personal computer. It was essentially an accounts receivable package that produced bills, insurance claims, and periodic reports. As various applications were developed for scheduling, electronic claims processing, and other business-oriented tasks, the hardware platforms expanded and the software applications became multitasking. It became necessary to exchange data between two or more workstations in or outside of the dental office.

Today, we have evolved from a single-user, single-tasking PC to the multiuser, multitasking, networked systems that allow rapid simultaneous processing and have large storage capabilities and integrated clinical applications (Fig 5-1). Increasingly, we view dental office automation from both a clinical as well as a business perspective. These networked systems have more favorable cost/performance ratios while providing an increasingly wider array of clinical services. The front office and the operatory are truly becoming integrated.

Operating System Software

There are two basic types of software: the *operating system* software and the *application* software. The application software performs the basic tasks, such as billing or imaging, that you want to accomplish. The operating system software, or "OS," is relatively transparent to the user and performs the background

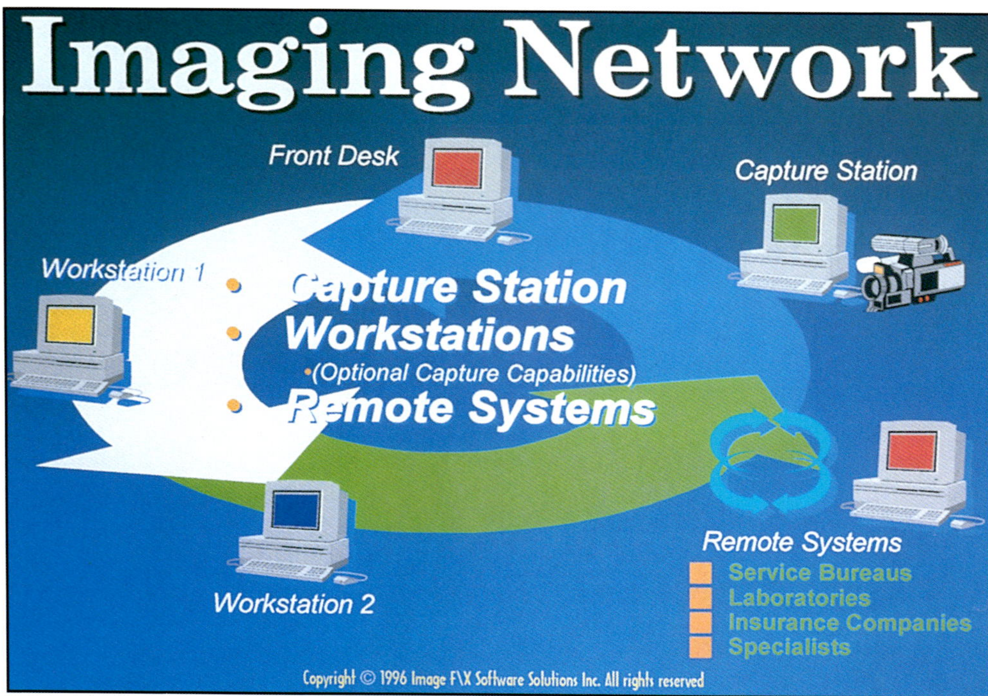

Fig 5-1 A typical dental office network configuration consists of a main server and interconnected client workstations that provide greater flexibility to the users. (Courtesy of Image FX Software Solutions Inc.)

housekeeping or traffic functions required to make the computer work. This means, for example, that it coordinates the activities of the keyboard, printer, and other "peripheral" devices, monitors the running of the workstations and different software packages, and maintains security and data integrity, as well as other technical functions. There is much written about the functions and merits of the different commercially available operating systems. It is wise to adhere to this basic principle when making a purchasing decision: buy industry standard, widely installed, well-maintained OS software.

The most popular operating systems today are industry standards such as MS/DOS, Windows, IBM OS/2, and Apple Macintosh OS, which are typically found in workstations, as well as UNIX and XENIX, which are used in "servers," or hubs, for multiple workstation environments. Microsoft has developed what may be the next generation of operating systems, Windows NT. It combines the attributes of both workstation and server operating systems and eliminates the need for two operating systems in a networked environment. All of these systems have graphical user interfaces that simplify user interaction with the application software. This means that they employ icons and other graphical images to simplify tasks for the nontechnical user. Because of the number of these popular operating systems already in use, more and better application software is constantly being written, upgraded, and maintained.

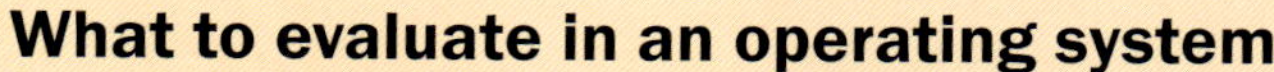

What to evaluate in an operating system

- Ease of use/graphical user interface
- Size of current user base
- Variety and suitability of application software available
- Maintenance and upgrade track record
- Speed and multitasking capability
- Ease of network connectivity
- Multilevel security

Application Software

Application software is the software that enables you to perform particular tasks. In addition to the traditional business functions, more dental application software is being developed and refined for clinical aspects of dentistry such as imaging and charting. Like all current software, clinical software must be easy to use and integrate with the business software in order to build and maintain an effective and useful database of patient information.

Software should also be modular and portable; that is, it should be able to be moved if you want to upgrade your hardware and/or replace some but not all of your current software applications. It is particularly important that all dental software adhere to both the computer industry standards as well as the emerging standards recommended by the American Dental Association's Dental Informatics Advisory Group (DIAG).[1] These standards are critical for the capture, storage, and transmission of clinical information such as patient images.

Requirements for system and application software

- Icon and menu driven/easy to use
- Fully integrateable with other appropriate software applications
- Appropriate for a network environment; not limited to a single-purpose, stand-alone system
- Adherent to basic computer industry standards
- Adherent to medical/dental standards (ADA and Computer-Based Oral Health Record[2])
- Well documented and supported
- Good history of periodic updates
- Implementation and training assistance
- Multilevel security
- Hardware-independent, modular software
- Compatible with anticipated storage requirements

Observe and analyze any potential system in a live, *appropriate* setting, not just in a sales situation.

Image Acquisition, Storage, and Retrieval

Imaging software can be separated into two specific modules, or functional areas: image acquisition, storage, and retrieval software, and image manipulation software. You should have the option to select a stand-alone imaging system that integrates seamlessly with the practice management system platform you currently use or may select in the future. Systems vendors usually welcome the opportunity to form a noncompetitive strategic alliance with each other, which results in a totally integrated automated platform for the dental office.

The imaging system should be able to acquire and store images from various sources and devices such as:

- Intraoral video cameras
- 35-mm cameras
- Scanners (including X-ray scanners)
- Digital cameras
- Video microscopes
- Extraoral video cameras
- Kodak Photo CD
- Digital radiography units
- VCRs
- Other computers

The system should also be able to translate images from one data format to another so that data exchange between dissimilar systems can be accomplished with little effort. This is especially useful when consulting with other specialists. To lessen the impact of hardware dependence and obsolescence, the software should adhere to computer industry standards that provide for portability. You should have the ability to capture an image, or a series of images, and store them automatically in a selected patient record without the need for redundant patient information data entry. And further, you should be able to make changes such as cropping, color adjustment, or rotating before saving the patient record.

Guidelines have been established for the patient record that conform to the Digital Imaging and Communications in Medicine (DICOM) standards for storing medical records and images.[3] This information is available in *The Computer-Based Oral Health Record* [2] and defines exactly what data must accompany each stored image. This information should be assigned automatically by the software.

Requirements for data storage

- Unique patient identifier
- Unique image identifier
- Time and date of image capture
- Image source
- Digitization method
- Horizontal and vertical dimensions
- Spatial scale
- Identifier for original vs manipulated image

Opening a patient record should be quick and easy; all of the information pertinent to a single patient should be available through the same command pathway. Ideally, when a patient's record is opened, the last full-face image is displayed (Fig 5-2). The next command should access the entire image file (Fig 5-3). If your practice is networked and fully integrated, a user can access, capture, and store data (within selected security parameters) from any workstation. This information should include all history and billing data as well as all automated clinical data and digitized images. All of this information should have a sorting capability based on various criteria such as image type, procedure, and patient age, for all manner of reporting and statistical analysis.

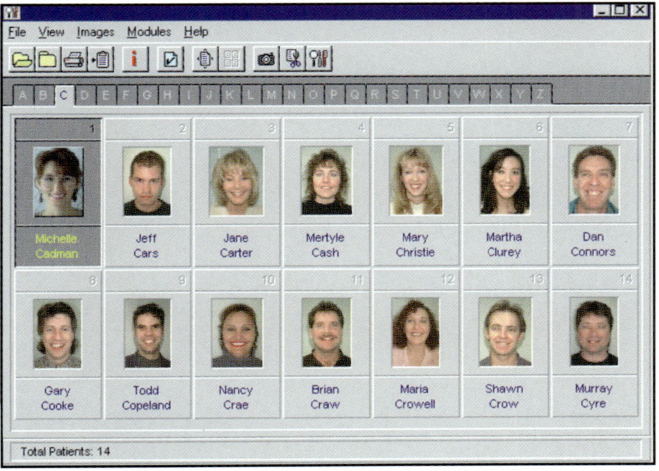

Fig 5-2 A patient's file is easy to identify when his or her last full-face image is displayed.

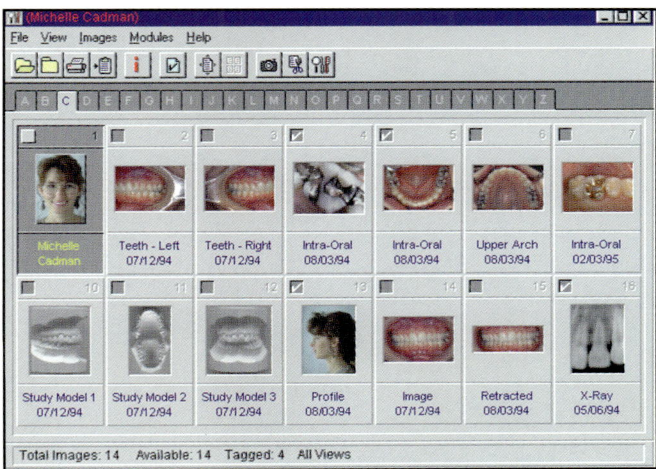

Fig 5-3 Ideally, to open a patient's file, the user should be able to simply click on the patient's image.

Once you have selected a patient image, you should be able to move it to another software application or module. For example, to modify an image, you should be able to select the cosmetic manipulation icon to display the tools for that task. Further, window sizing for each image should be automatic and the image displayed on a blank background with its unique label and date. Avoid systems with floating image windows, which place a scalable image on top of an active application, as they are difficult to work with.

Memory and compression/decompression. The image resolutions and magnifications necessary for precise diagnostic evaluations of any clinical situation require a substantial amount of computer memory and storage capacity. The good news is that the cost of memory and disk storage devices continuously decrease while the capacities increase.

The image acquisition software should be designed to automatically recognize whenever more memory or storage is added. The system should also be capable of storing and retrieving captured images quickly for real-time review on high-resolution monitors, printing to high-resolution printing devices, transmitting to remote sites for consultations, as well as providing for image manipulation.

If data compression is necessary for conservation of disk storage or data transmission, it is most important that the compression/decompression software result in no image degradation in the process. Data transmission and reception also require that the decompression algorithms (mathematical formulas) interpret multiple standard image formats such as JPEG, GIF, and TIFF. The image storage system should be designed to archive images with informational tags that provide for patient, doctor, date, and other cross-referencing data.

Requirements for image acquisition, storage, and retrieval systems

- Expandable memory and storage capacity
- Rapid data compression/decompression functions
- Zero image degradation with decompression
- LAN access from all available workstations
- Multiple image format capability

The key to system selection is to carefully research and monitor the direction of industry standards. For example, years ago Sony developed a proprietary Beta-format videotape system that was higher quality than the competition, VHS, which utilized an open standard format. However, because of the proprietary nature of the Sony system, few tapes were manufactured, and the public ultimately chose VHS. Since many manufacturers were producing an abundant supply of VHS products, the costs were lowered.

The Apple is another example of a proprietary architecture. Much less software is developed for Apple computers than for the IBM (Intel) PC. Also, IBM-compatible hardware and software can be acquired from many sources, thus lowering the cost and maximizing flexibility. Unless an imaging system has a key feature that no other system has, and you feel absolutely that you must have it, avoid proprietary vendor systems that restrict you from taking advantage of technology advances from multiple sources.

When planning for an imaging system, you may want to work with an independent consultant who has experience with the technical aspects. In any event, it is best not to decide to acquire a system based solely on the information supplied by the salesman or vendor.

Image Manipulation

A dentist or imaging specialist can simulate such procedures as bleaching, veneering and bonding, crown and bridge, crown lengthening, orthodontics, cosmetic contouring, or periodontal soft-tissue changes (Fig 5-4). The various types of simulations are covered in depth in Chapter 8. However, the key to success with cosmetic simulation is easy-to-use image manipulation software. Earlier versions of imaging tools performed only one function at a time and required advanced skill to create a good cosmetic simulation. In newer software, the graphics tablet and pen have given way to the standard computer mouse for ease, multifunctionality, and greater accuracy.

Once the dentist or imaging specialist has made the image enhancements specified by the patient or treatment plan, the new image can be saved. The computer should automatically identify the image as an altered version of the original. A printed copy of any image, with the associated tag identifiers, should be able to be produced at any time during the manipulation process (Fig 5-5).

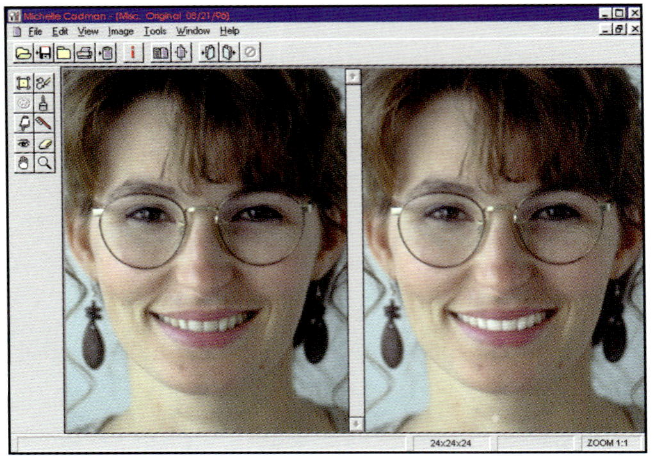

a

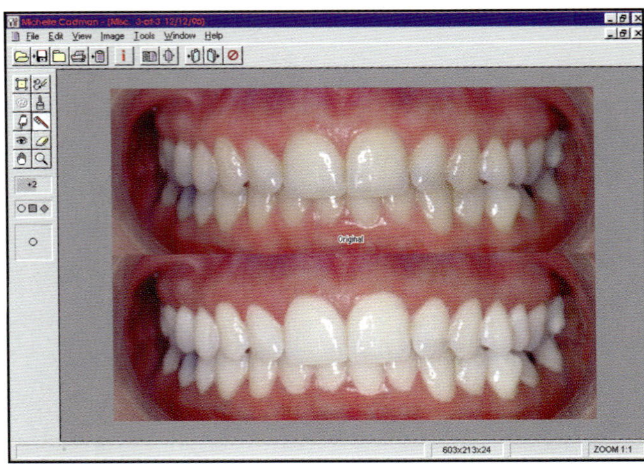

b

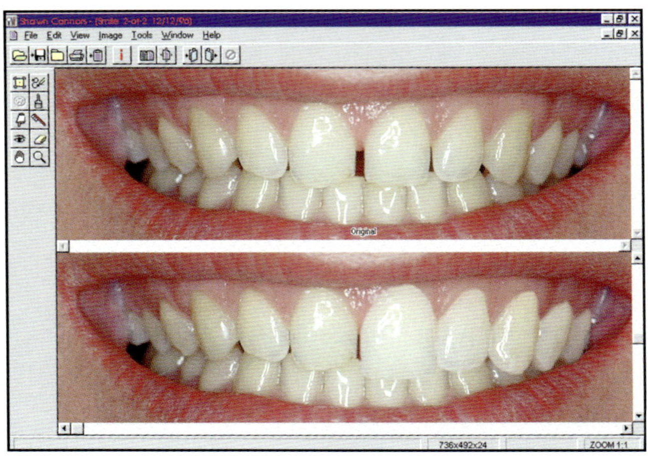

c

Fig 5-4a to c *The software tools should not only be simple, but they should enable the operator to make the required changes automatically, whether lightening teeth (a and b) or experimenting with different tooth forms and incisal edge positions prior to laminate veneers (c).*

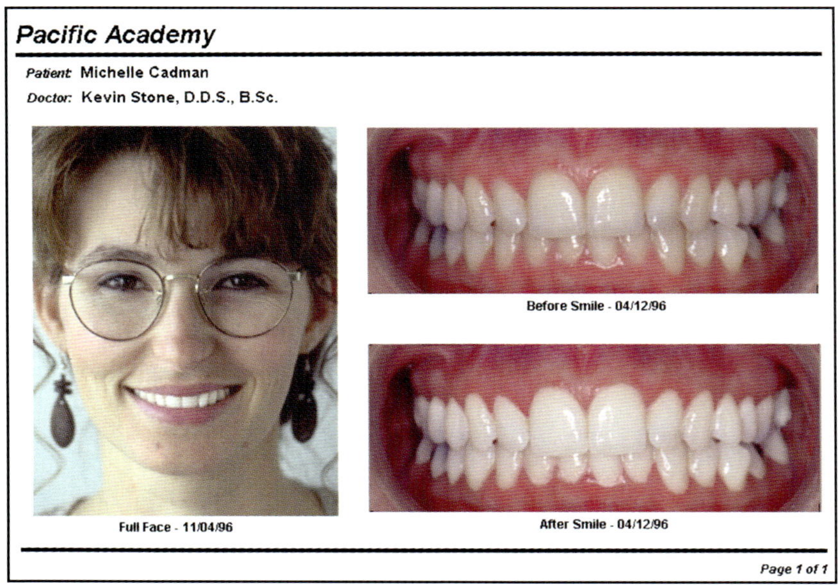

Fig 5-5 *An important key feature of image simulation software is its ability to output to a photo-realistic digital printer or another digital output device.*

Requirements for image manipulation software

- Easy to use (a high level of technical or graphical skills should not be necessary for a dental cosmetic simulation)
- Multifunctional tools
- The ability to work on the image simulation while viewing the original, untouched image
- The ability of the bleaching tool to not bleach the gingiva and not require the outlining of each tooth
- The ability to manipulate the color beyond lightening and darkening, using tints to match and blend tooth colors
- The ability to include or remove teeth from image to image
- The ability to outline and reshape a unique region of the smile rather than erasing an unwanted bilateral alteration.
- The ability to annotate unique descriptions on the image
- Progressive save capability to eliminate a total restart for intermediate mistakes or changes
- The ability to paint various levels of tooth texture
- The ability to make and display measurements of select areas of the image
- Library of smile images (smile bank); the smiles must be integrated with the face, not "pasted" onto it
- The ability to blend the image with varying intensities
- The ability to pull (or drag) a region of the image using various densities of the original image
- The ability to stretch, pull, flip, proportionately size, and move portions of the image
- The ability to print to any digital output device

Finally, be aware of software and software components that are "in development," not "live" in a practice environment. Consider it vaporware until you see it work.

References

1. Jones L. Dental Informatics. Integrating Technology into the Dental Environment. New York: Springer-Verlag, 1992.
2. Eisner J, Chasteen JE, Schleyer T, et al. The Computer-Based Oral Health Record. The AADS Consortium for Clinical Information Systems, 1993.
3. Digital Imaging and Communications in Medicine (DICOM). Washington: National Electrical Manufacturers Association, 1993.

The Imaging *Appointment*

6

Computer imaging is a powerful way to communicate to patients what can be accomplished in dentistry using advanced technology. Fully realizing the potential of your system, though, requires careful planning.

The equipment should be set up in a manner that not only facilitates its use but also encourages patients to relax and participate (See Chapter 12 for specific suggestions). Be aware that a successful imaging consultation requires that you match your knowledge of dentistry with a comfortable expertise in the skills of computer imaging. The more you use your system, the more proficient you will become.

Preparing the Patient

Most imaging appointments are for esthetic consultation and treatment planning. Ask your patients to prepare by looking through magazines and collecting photos of smiles and teeth that they find attractive. These images can give you and your patient a starting point for discussing and imaging various esthetic options.

As you and your patients evaluate treatment options, make it clear that the computer-generated image cannot show *exactly* how proposed changes will look. It is only a two-dimensional approximation of a predicted result. Point out that, in reality, treating living tissues is not an exact science, and the three-dimensional result may vary from the two-dimensional image.

It can also be helpful if patients bring in photographs of their own smiles taken before any undesirable changes took place. If the photographs span several years, their teeth may show changes such as incisal edge wear, tooth movement, or loss that may have left an unattractive space. Imaging will enable you to show your patients how these changes can be reversed.

Because the objective of this appointment is cosmetic enhancement, ask patients to come to the imaging session looking their best. Women who normally wear makeup should do so for the consultation. Also, patients should wear a flattering color. White clothing near the face should be avoided, however, because video cameras tend to compensate for the brightness by shutting down the electronic camera iris, resulting in a grainy image (Fig 6-1a). Patients who arrive wearing white may be given a blue drape to place over their shoulders (Fig 6-1b).

While advance preparation for an imaging session is desirable, it is not mandatory. There will be many instances when a routine hygiene appointment leads directly to an imaging consultation. By all means, seize these opportunities when they arise. Even without preparation, patients who are curious about the potential for esthetic changes will be receptive to an imaging demonstration of how dentistry might improve their appearance.

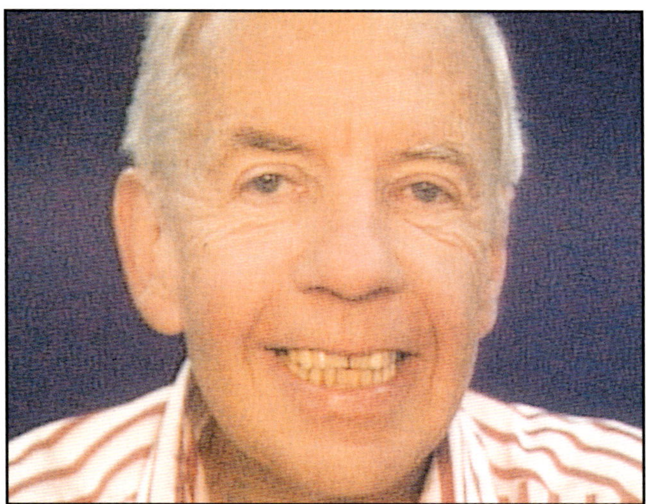

Fig 6-1a *Light-colored clothing causes grainy images.*

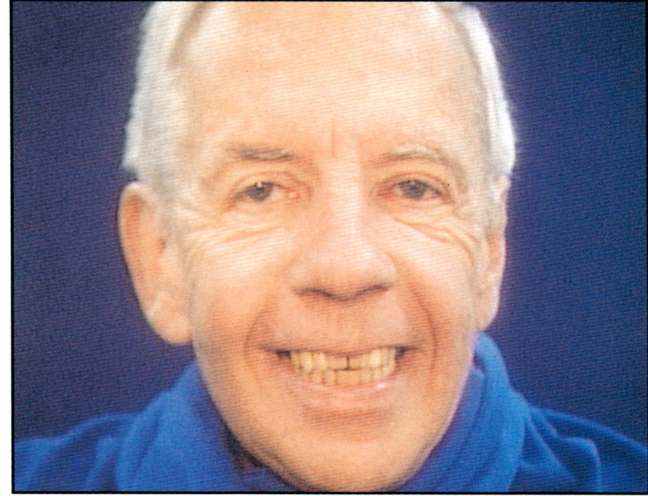

Fig 6-1b *A royal blue cloth drape can be used to cover any light-colored clothing.*

What the Camera Reveals

If you want to help your patients receive the most benefit from an imaging consultation, you should first understand some of the psychology underlying the process.

For example, when we see ourselves in the mirror, a mole on the left side appears to be on the right side of the face. Not so in a photographic image (Fig 6-2a). One reason computer imaging is so effective is that it allows patients to see themselves as others see them (Fig 6-2b). This has proven to be an important key to unlocking the sophisticated mechanisms of the subconscious mind that keep patients from acknowledging and accepting certain aspects of their appearance. This concept, identified by a research team at Envision International in Indianapolis, Indiana, is called *subliminal esthetic mapping.* The name suggests the actual mechanism: We tend to block out those aspects of our physical image that we perceive as unattractive and feel we either cannot or will not change.

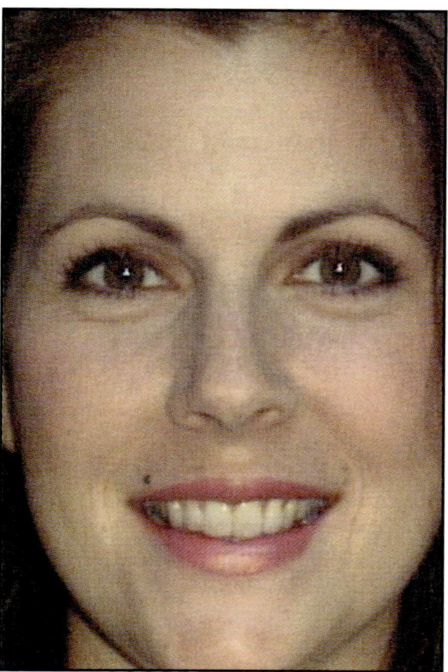

Fig 6-2a *This 35-mm photograph shows the patient's mirror image.*

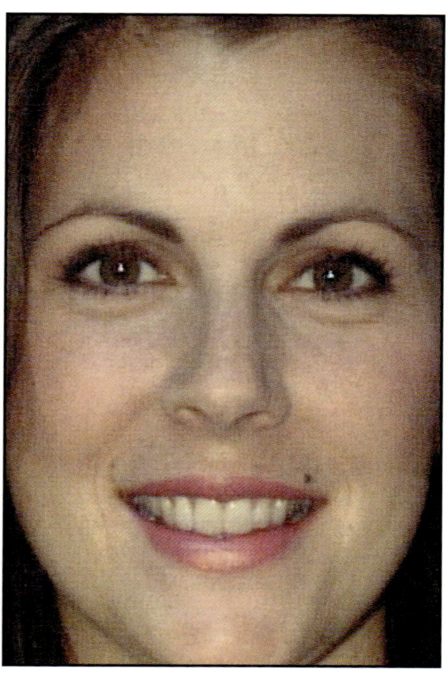

Fig 6-2b *This computer image shows the patient's true self, not a mirror image.*

When patients first see themselves on the imaging screen, they typically remark that they were unaware of how they appear to others. In the moments that follow that realization, patients begin pointing out nuances of their appearance that they have always found bothersome, but have learned to accept, or even hide, through a variety of mechanisms such as restrained lip positioning. A patient with vertical maxillary excess who would normally expose several millimeters of gingival tissue when laughing may pose the smile instinctively with the inferior aspect of the upper lip resting right at the cervical margin (Fig 6-3). Is such a patient bothered by a gummy smile? Absolutely. The elaborate subconscious mechanisms developed over time to mask it are proof of its negative impact on the patient's self-image.

By correctly diagnosing such behaviors through imaging, we can address these issues and offer solutions. It is not uncommon for esthetic dentistry to trigger additional unexpected changes that further enhance the patient's self-image. Once they finish dental treatment, patients often go on to lose weight, restyle their hair, improve a relationship, receive a promotion, or even launch a new career. What made the difference? One interpretation is that solving an esthetic problem helped them gain the confidence and self-esteem they needed to positively project themselves and become successful—a real, very powerful effect that transcends the traditional view of dentistry.

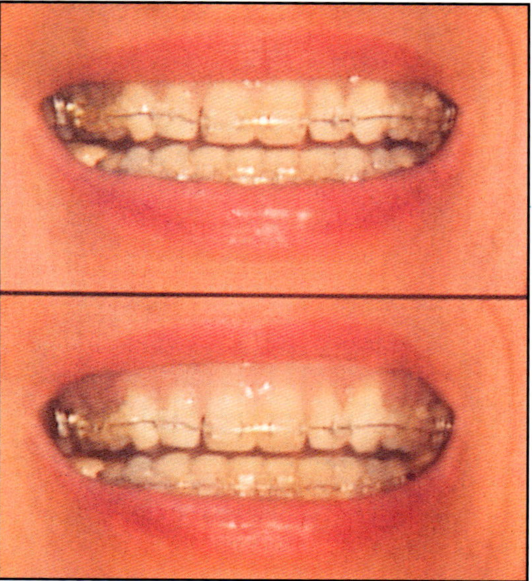

Fig 6-3 *Top, This patient has adopted a forced half smile to hide her gummy smile. Bottom, Be sure to capture the patient's true full smile.*

Such dramatic results aside, you should be prepared for the surprise or dismay your patients may experience when they first see their image. Put them at ease by explaining that they are accustomed to seeing themselves in the mirror, which provides a reversed thus different image. Also, while the face in life is constantly moving and changing, the two-dimensional image is frozen in time so you can analyze the smile without the distraction of movement. Even the best diagnostic picture probably won't be the most flattering. The camera sees all and exacerbates any disparities (which is why film and television stars spend so much time in makeup before they face the camera). Your reassurances can help patients through the initial shock of facing their images.

Even the best diagnostic picture probably won't be the most flattering.

To encourage patient interest and participation, it is best to perform image changes in their presence. The wizardry of the computer simulations usually impresses patients and they will often talk about it with their friends, family, and coworkers. This type of internal marketing can be quite beneficial to your practice. Bleaching, cosmetic contouring, or simple tooth replacement are all easily imaged within a few minutes while your patient is watching. Sometimes, however, you may need time to study the photos and try possible treatment options; in that case, you may want to ask the patient to return at a later time.

Above all, encourage your patients to relax and have fun with the imaging process. Aim for a free exchange of ideas—yours and the patient's—and see how different options might work. This interactive discussion is essential for obtaining the best result.

Obtaining Images

The best esthetic results are obtained by starting with accurate and clear computer images. Digitized video images are the current standard and will probably continue to be so. Thirty-five millimeter cameras still provide the most detailed images, and these images can be scanned into your computer or placed onto a Photo CD. In this case, however, your imaging cannot be done at the consultation visit since the 35-mm slides need to be developed and stored on a Photo CD.

Table 6-1 lists and references various images that may be needed, depending on the type of changes you want to show. Take as many or as few images as you will need to document and explain the diagnosis.[1]

Table 6-1

Full Face

Frontal

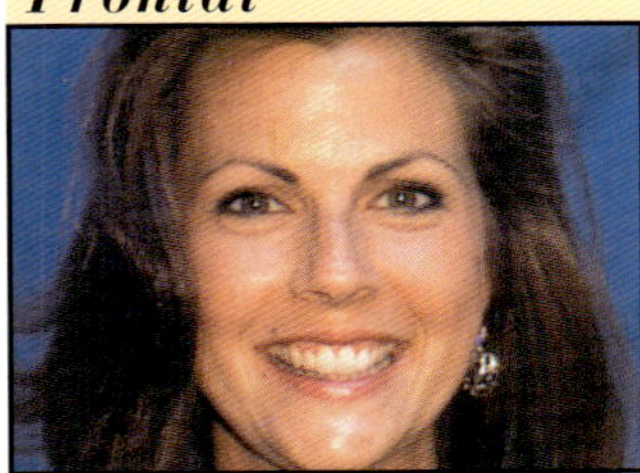

Fig 6-4a Maximum smile. This is often the image used for your changes.

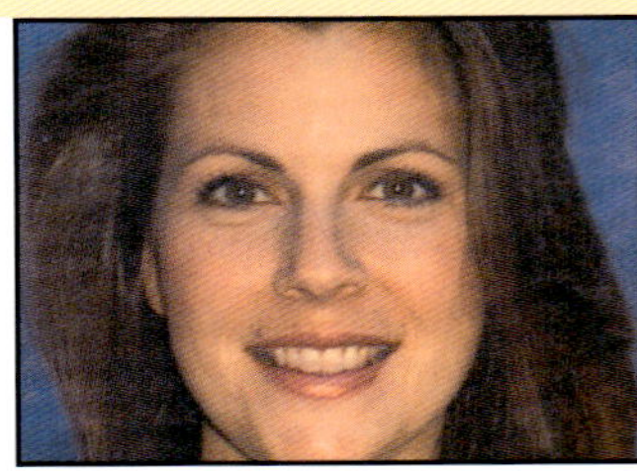

Fig 6-4b Smile. The patient with a normal, relaxed smile.

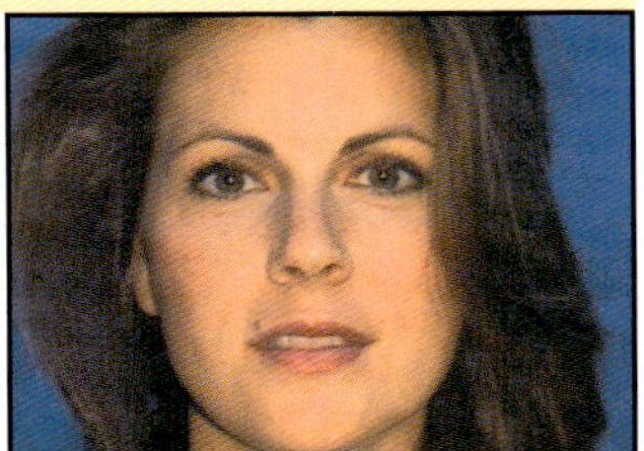

Fig 6-4c Lips in repose. The patient's face with the lips in a relaxed position and the mandible at the vertical dimension of rest.

Oblique

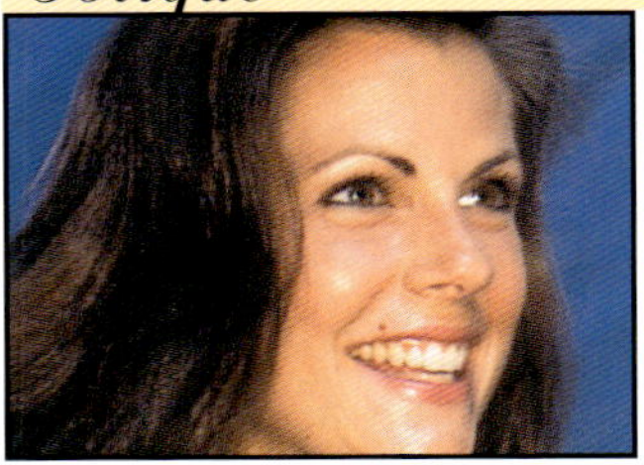

Fig 6-5a Maximum smile. Your patients can now see what others see when they laugh.

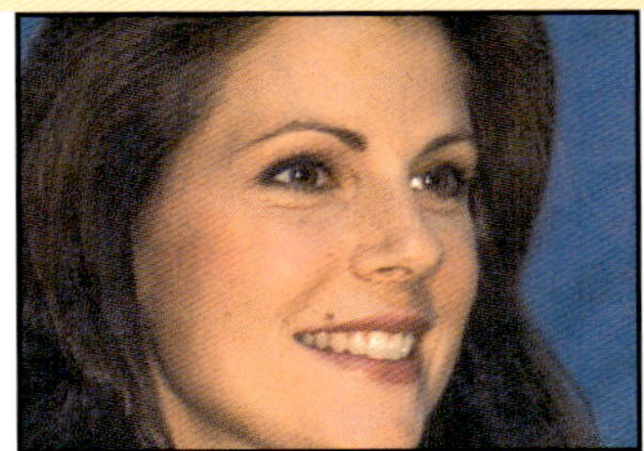

Fig 6-5b Smile. This view is especially helpful to show patients how many of their posterior teeth show when they smile.

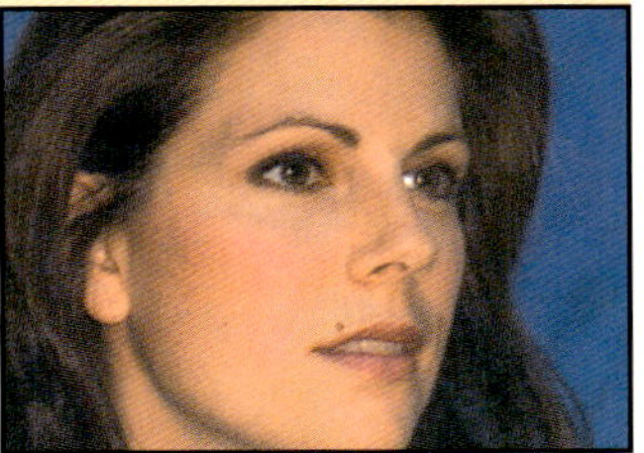

Fig 6-5c Lips in repose. The speaking line or incisal edges are seen in relation to the lipline in this view.

Lateral

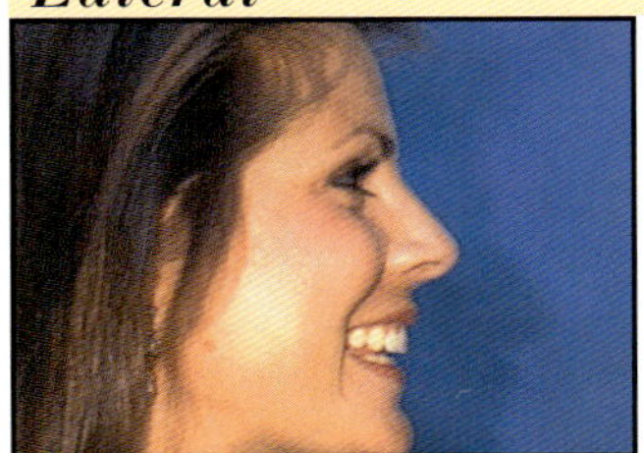

Fig 6-6a Maximum smile. This angle is easily used in your before and after images.

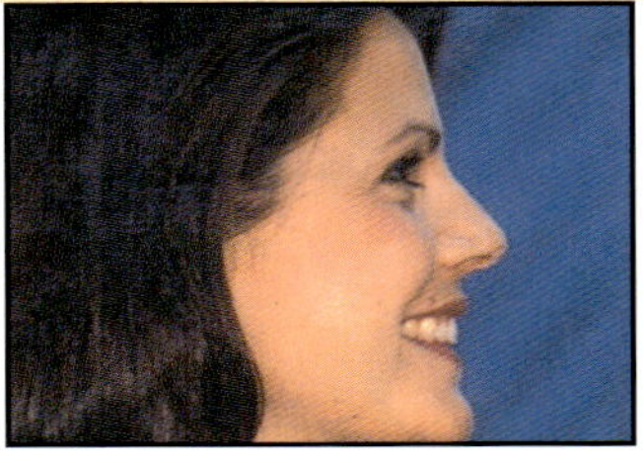

Fig 6-6b Smile. The patient rarely sees this side view, which reveals the relative angle of the anterior teeth in relation to the lips and face, and is helpful from both an orthodontic and orthognathic perspective.

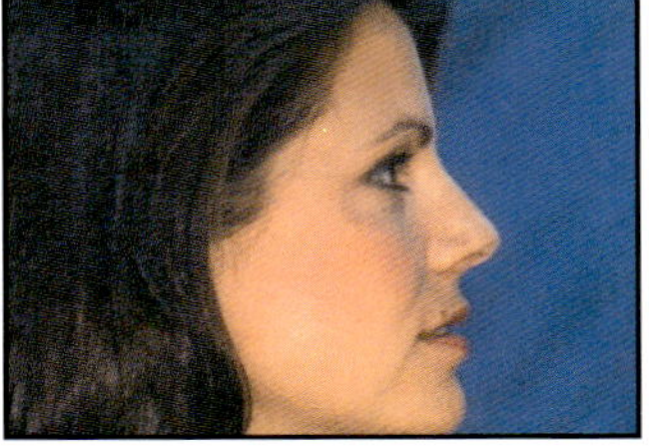

Fig 6-6c Lips in repose (profile) allow easy evaluation of the patient's profile including nose, chin, and anterior tooth and lip positions.

Three-Quarter Face

(take when this view is necessary to show dramatic improvement that can only be seen from this view)

Frontal

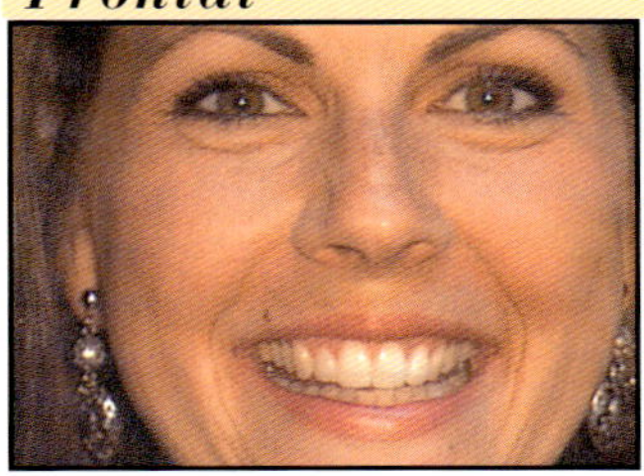

Fig 6-7a Maximum smile with teeth parted. Helpful for the patient to see in detail how their teeth and smile relate to the lower portion of their face.

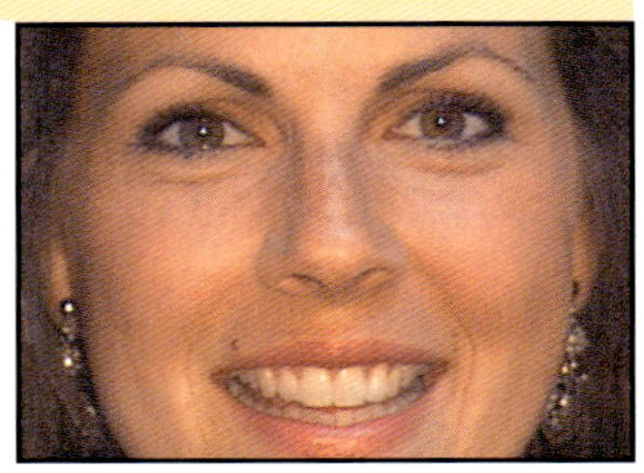

Fig 6-7b Smile. This view helps patients to focus on any incisal edge discrepancies and lip imperfections.

Oblique

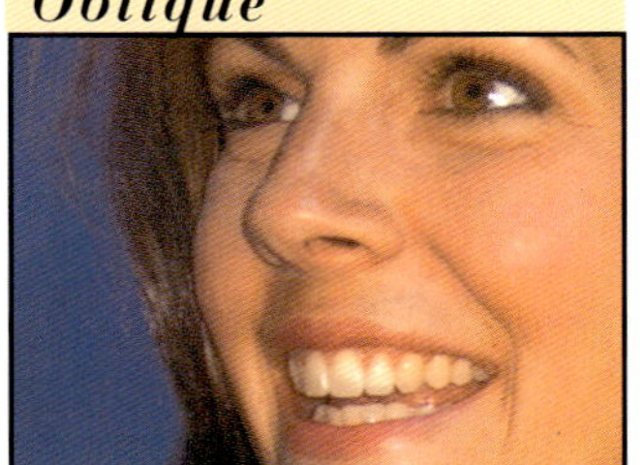

Fig 6-7c Maximum smile. You and your patient can evaluate what your patient never sees—the side view.

Lateral

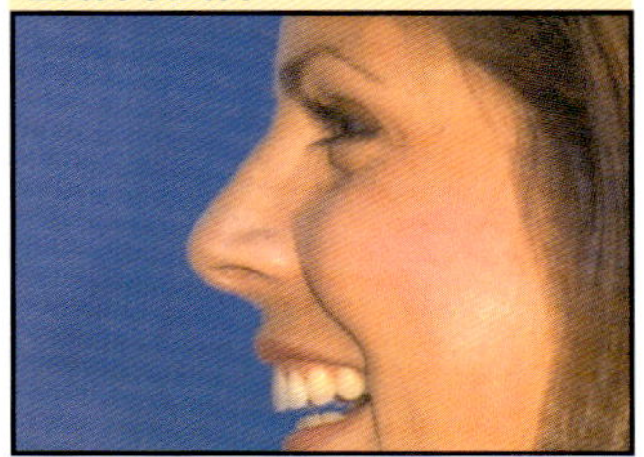

Fig 6-7d Maximum smile. Angulations of the teeth in relation to the lower half of the face are easily evaluated.

Close-Up Smile

Frontal

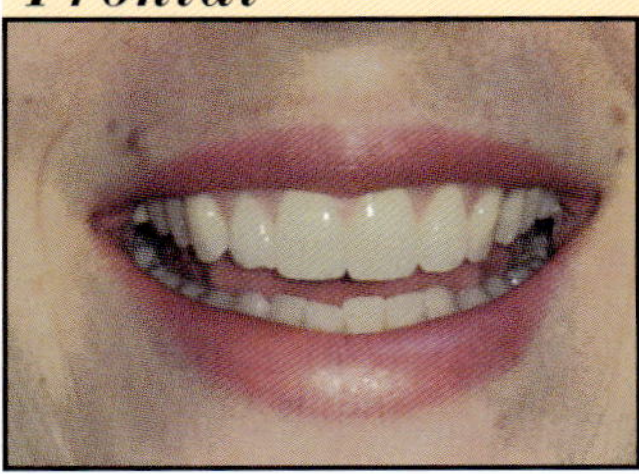

Fig 6-8a Maximum smile with teeth parted. An essential view showing the incisal edges, this is the single most-used view for making computer alterations.

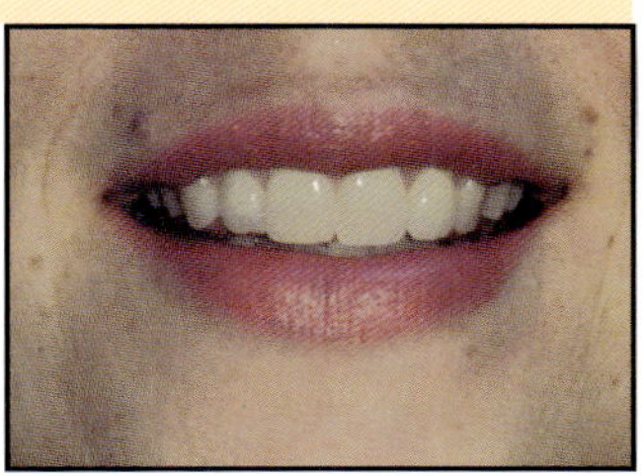

Fig 6-8b Slight smile. Helpful for viewing the buccal vestibules, speaking or smile line, and other features of the smile.

Oblique

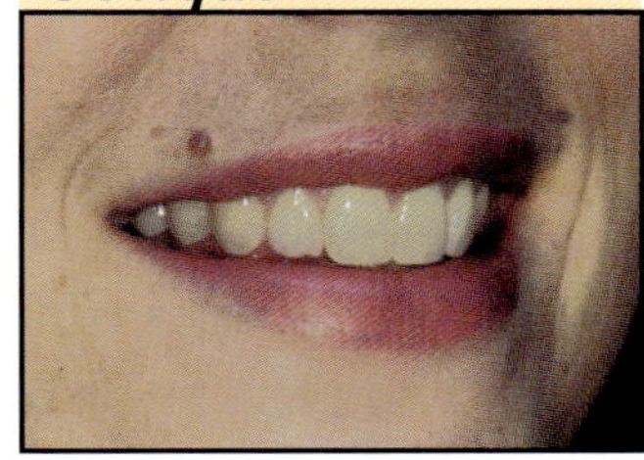

Fig 6-8c A close-up showing the patient what others see; also helpful in diagnosing problems in the silhouette form of the teeth.

Lateral

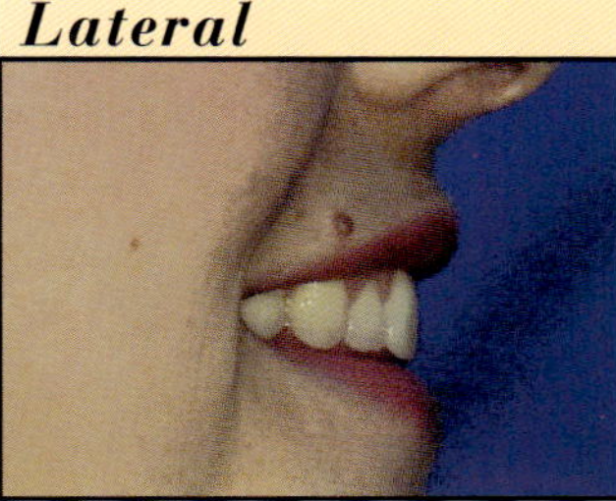

Fig 6-8d Profile. Helpful in diagnosing skeletal deformities and orthodontic problems.

Lips Retracted

Frontal

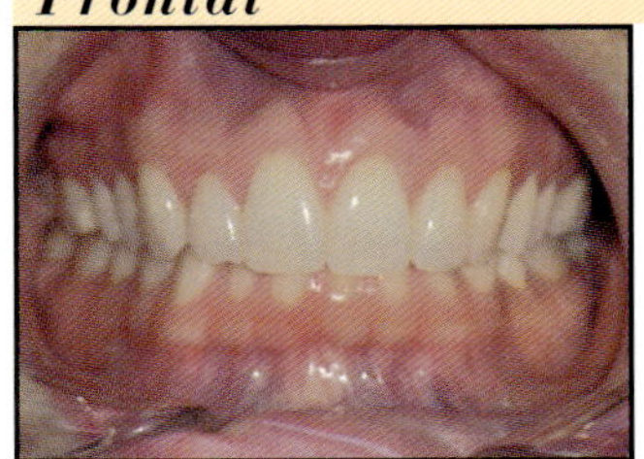

Fig 6-9a Centric occlusion and centric relation. Useful for documenting pretreatment occlusal relationships.

Fig 6-9b Teeth apart. Provides a clear view of the incisal edges.

Oblique

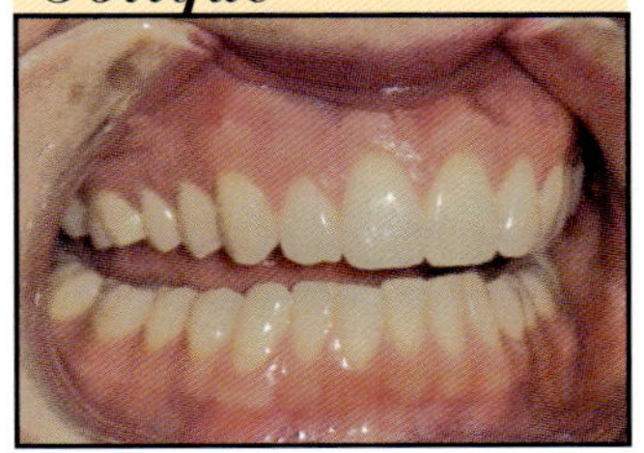

Fig 6-9c Teeth apart. A good angle to demonstrate occlusal problems such as wear.

Lateral

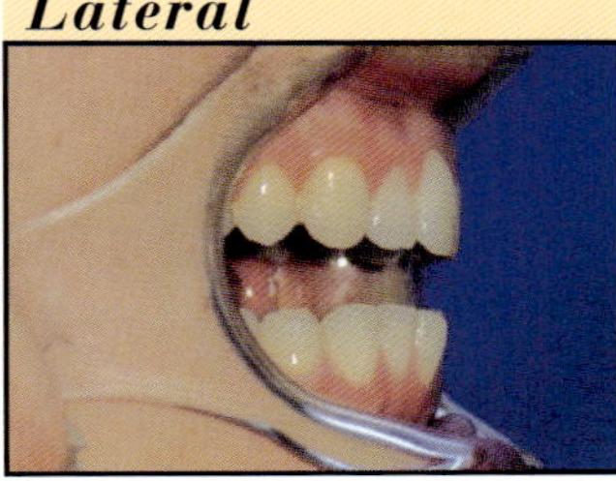

Fig 6-9d Teeth apart. Orthodontists and orthognathic surgeons use this view for certain analyses.

Arch Form

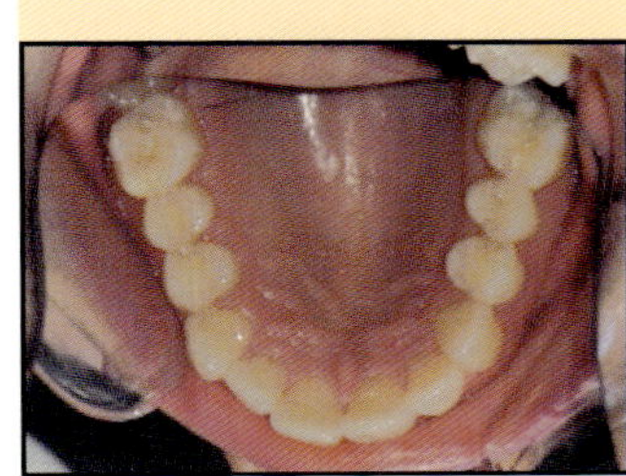

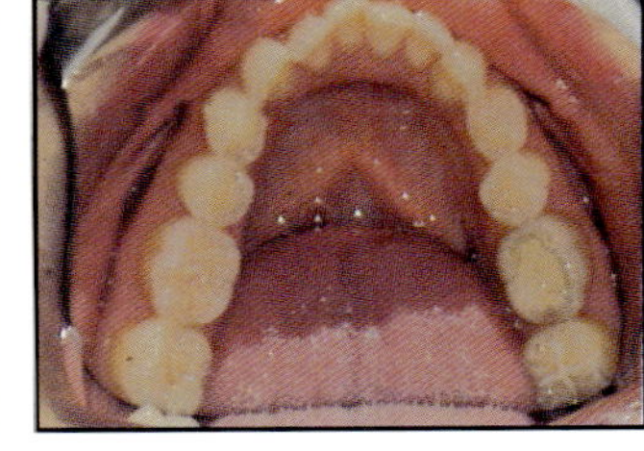

Fig 6-10a and **b** Occlusal views of the maxilla and mandible are both useful for pretreatment documentation.

Background

Use a seamless, one-color background for all of your imaging to enable you to move parts from one image to another with ease. This will also eliminate background distractions in the room.

A solid, medium-blue background will give good contrast and be pleasing to the eye. The wall may be painted, or you can hang a blue cloth curtain behind the patient, taking care to smooth out any wrinkles and folds. Other options include a large posterboard from an art supply store or a blue, seamless paper backdrop used by photographers. If you are using a software system with sizing grids, the need for a consistent background color may be eliminated.

Lighting

Ideally, the imaging area should be lit exclusively with color-corrected artificial light. Because the quality of natural light changes during the course of the day, it is best to exclude daylight from the imaging area (Fig 6-11a and b). Ambient light should be controlled by a rheostat (dimmer) so that the light can be altered as needed depending on the patient's skin tones, hair, and clothing.

Imaging systems are equipped with their own light source that correctly illuminates the patient. But no matter how carefully you try to control it, the light may vary from one image to the next, even those taken in close succession. One system has a unique "posttreatment" mode that allows you to compare and

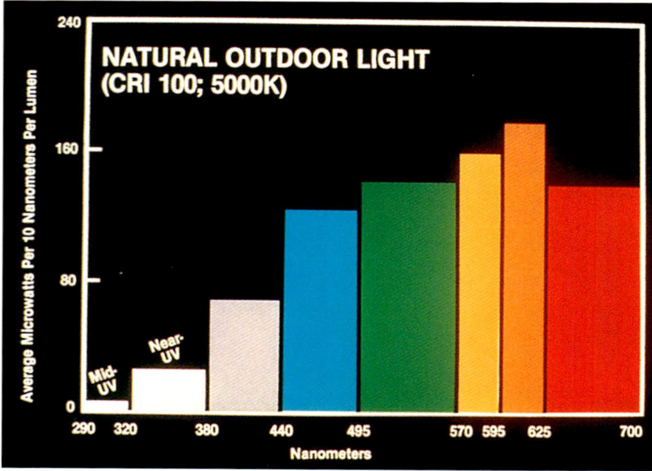

Fig 6-11a The color spectrum of natural light.

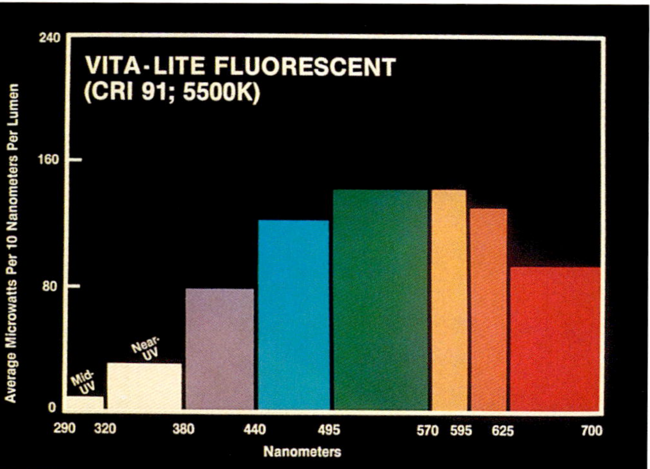

Fig 6-11b Use color-corrected bulbs, such as the Vita-Lite fluorescent tubes, in your imaging room. (Courtesy of Duro-test, Corp.)

match the color and brightness of an existing image with current conditions. This is also useful when obtaining both the close-up images, which show fine detail, and the full-face images. Because close-up images have a different degree of luminance (they may appear brighter or darker) than full-face images of the same subject, you should adjust the light accordingly if you intend to combine portions of different views. New software color correction packages and portable extraoral cameras allow you to capture images anywhere in the office without the limitations of special lighting requirements.

Chair Position

Select a chair that is comfortable for the patient and provides easy adjustments to allow for the proper angle between patient and camera. If the patient is in a strained position, it will be difficult for them to give you a relaxed smile. If you plan to use a dental chair to image your patients, you can remove the head rest to allow you to more easily alter the head position.

Patient Position

Begin by having your patient look straight at the camera, then suggest slight head movements to obtain the exact head position on the monitor necessary for the desired picture. Your goal in an imaging session is to obtain one or more images that will be useful to the diagnostic process. Images must be sharp, the color as true as possible, and the position of the head correct. Understand that it is not easy or natural to smile with the head perfectly straight and that people tend to tilt their heads when smiling. Explain to the patient that most faces are asymmetrical; with the head held straight, it will be easier to see asymmetries and determine how to create the most harmonious smile.

Keep the patient in the same position while taking full-face and close-up images in close succession.

In addition to obtaining an image of the patient's smile, you may also want to pose the patient while he or she is grimacing or retracting the lips. This will enable you to see more clearly the shape of the arch, the shape of the lips in relation to the teeth, the teeth in relation to the smile, and the smile in relation to the face. Profiles or oblique angles of the face or smile may also be useful to focus on the shape of a certain tooth, the color of individual teeth, and the relation of teeth to each other. Retractors may be required to show all of the teeth and gums in a single image.

Keep the patient in the same position while taking full-face and close-up images in close succession, especially if the close-up smile will be altered and used to create the full-face "after" image. This will help ensure that the face and the angle of the smile do not change from one image to the next. Sometimes, if the full-face image is captured close enough, you can make simple changes to the teeth without using a close-up image, but this is the exception to the rule. The challenge of showing subtle but important nuances of esthetics in smile design is accomplished more easily with a close-up view of the smile.

When making your photograph, the patient's occlusal plane should be parallel to the floor from both the front and side views. The camera should be level with the patient's head; aiming the camera up or down tends to distort the teeth. Pose the patient with the incisal edges slightly parted and silhouetted against the black shadows of the intraoral cavity. This will help to delineate the shape of the teeth. Also, the overlap of the maxillary anterior dentition may obscure unattractive, irregular incisal edge relationships on the mandibular incisors or other esthetic problems.

If unusual features are present, capture them close up.

You should make an image of the patient's maximum smile showing the lips at their highest point. While this can sometimes be difficult to capture, it can usually be achieved by injecting humor (eg, asking your patient to say "belly-button"), prompting the patient to laugh. This may even require two people—one to help make the patient laugh, and the other to capture the image. Be sure to keep the patient's hands away from the mouth. This is a common masking technique among people who are uncomfortable or embarrassed by their smiles.

Many esthetic problems are most evident from the lateral view, yet patients are usually most concerned with their smiles from canine to canine. However, most smiles extend as far as the mesial of the first molar and often to the distal of the second molar. Patients who fail to understand this situation may compromise their treatment plan by addressing only the six anterior teeth. Capturing and modifying the profile view of the patient's full smile can help in these cases. To capture the profile, turn the chair to the side. A swivel chair simplifies this and can also help you maintain correct height and angular position. Have the patient hold this position with the mouth either closed or smiling as desired.

If unusual features are present, capture them close up. Use the close-up lens for diastemas or mottled enamel.

Additional Tools

If you do not intend to modify the images on the computer yourself, a checklist is a useful way to specify changes for the imaging technician (Form 6-1).

Form 6-2 is a question-and-answer handout provided for you to copy and reprint with your own practice's heading. This handout may help answer many of your patient's questions and concerns about computerized imaging.

Computer Imaging Checklist

DDS/DMD ______________________
Imaging technician ______________________
Treatment coordinator ______________________
Date ______________________

Doctor check ______________________
Patient check ______________________
Prints ______________________
Slides ______________________
Laser ______________________

Name ______________________
Address ______________________
____
Phone ______________________
Home Business

Patient's main concern ______________________
____

Proposed Changes

Teeth

Bleaching ______________________
Cosmetic contouring ______________________
Smile line ______________________
Laminates/bonding ______________________
Restorations ______________________
Tissue surgery (type) ______________________
Orthodontics ______________________

Face

Eyes ______________________
Nose ______________________
Chin ______________________
Profile ______________________
Other ______________________

Hair

Color ______________________
Length ______________________
Other ______________________

Other

Makeup ______________________
____
____

Consultants/specialists

Plastic surgery ______________________
Orthodontics ______________________
Orthognathic surgery ______________________
Other ______________________
____

Comments

____
____
____
____
____

Form 6-1

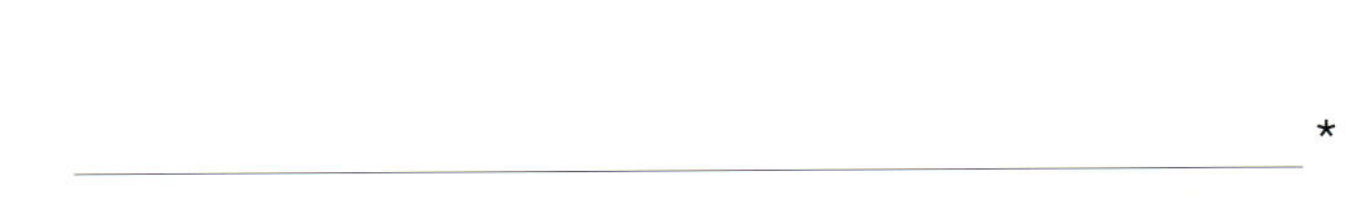

Computerized Imaging

Computerized imaging allows you to "see" your options for changing the way you look before you actually start any treatment. The following information may answer some of your questions.

Q: ***What should I expect during the consultation?***

A: During your consultation appointment, we'll take one or more pictures of you. With these and the computer, we'll be able to change the way you look on-screen, so you can see how different procedures can improve your appearance.

Depending on the complexity of your case and your own preference, you may watch while we work on your image or return at a later time to view and discuss the computer-imaged treatment proposal. Either way, feel free to tell us what you do and don't like about the way you look now or the changes you see on-screen. We want you to be comfortable and confident about any treatment before you make a commitment.

Q: ***Is there anything I should do to prepare for the consultation?***

A: Absolutely! We'd like you to take some time to look through magazines and collect photos of smiles and teeth you think are attractive. Please bring these to your appointment because they'll help us understand what you like or expect.

It's also a good idea to bring photos of yourself—ones that show your smile and teeth. If you can, bring a mix of recent and older pictures, so we can see how your teeth have changed over time.

Q: ***Why do I have to smile so widely?***

A: We'd like you to practice an exaggerated smile. Try to show as much of your teeth and gums as you can. We may take some pictures of your exaggerated smile to plan the details of your dental treatment. We understand that you might feel self-conscious posing like this, but it helps us to know the limits of your smile to plan your treatment. Unfortunately, the best diagnostic photos usually aren't the most flattering ones. Try to have a sense of humor about it and don't worry—nobody will see the pictures except you and the members of your treatment team.

Form 6-2

*Insert your practice name and telephone number.

Q: ***How accurate are computer-modified images?***

A: An excellent question. We use the computer to help you visualize how proposed changes will affect your appearance, but the computer image is not a literal representation of the results. Because the actual changes will involve living tissue, no one can predict with absolute certainty how your treatment will change your looks. So consider the computer image an *approximation*, based on our experience and knowledge, of how you will look after treatment.

Q: ***What should I wear to the appointment?***

A: Because the objective of this appointment is to enhance your appearance, we'd like you to come to the imaging session looking your best. If you normally wear makeup, please wear it for your consultation. Also, wear a color that looks good on you and flatters your skin tone and hair. Please avoid white or a very light color close to your face; the bright reflections can overwhelm the camera's automatic exposure feature and make it difficult to get accurate pictures of you.

Q: ***Is there anything else I should know before my appointment?***

A: Two things. First, tell us if you're interested in making changes besides the ones you may have already discussed with us. Maybe there's something else about your appearance that you'd like to change—a "gummy" smile, for instance, or the shape of your nose. Even if you aren't planning an immediate change, it could help us plan for your long-term dental treatment if we know that there are other aspects of your appearance you might like to change. If you want, we can also show you on the computer how you might look with a chin implant, a brow lift, a different hair style—you name it. The great thing about computer imaging is that it's a no-risk way to explore your esthetic options.

Finally, come to your imaging appointment prepared to relax and have fun. We look forward to seeing you!

If you have any other questions before your appointment, please call during office hours.

Reference

1. Goldstein RE. Esthetics in Dentistry, ed 2, vol I. Toronto: Decker, 1998.

The Three-Step *Analysis*

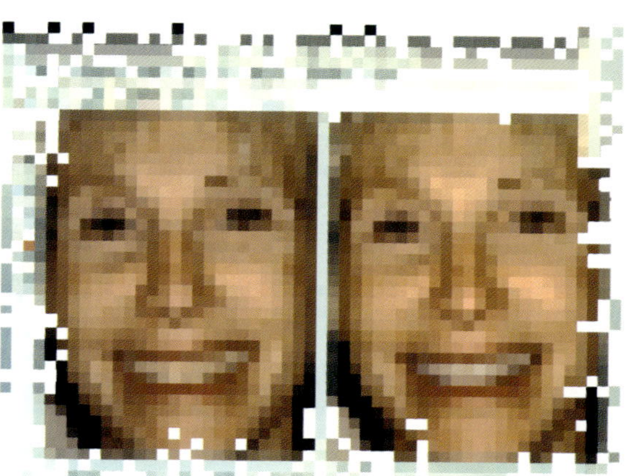

7

Jonathan Levine, DMD

Twenty years ago Peter Dawson said, "If you know where you are and you know where you want to go, getting there is easy." Here lies the key to successful results in esthetic dentistry. A clear, systematic approach to esthetic problems is required. First, the problem(s) must be identified and then the solution visualized. Appropriate techniques can be chosen to achieve the visualized solution. It is important that the dentist define early in the process what can and cannot be achieved. A structured, systematic approach eliminates the problem of technique-driven diagnoses.

Most dentists diagnose esthetic problems using the traditional tools of radiography and clinical examination. They then make decisions based on their own view of esthetics. Clinicians' ideas about facial esthetics, however, may not coincide with patients' perceptions and expectations; this is where many problems begin.

A structured approach promotes communication and therefore facilitates successful outcomes. First, it is important to develop a therapeutic mind-set, a systematic approach to esthetic problems. This systematic approach consists of identifying the problem and visualizing the solution with both the patient and the technician. Identifying the problem requires a three-step analysis[1] of the patient's esthetic concerns; this includes the esthetic evaluation form, computer imaging, and a diagnostic cast and wax-up. Information compiled from a combination of words, pictures, and models can minimize the possibility of misunderstanding amongst the dental team or between the dental team and the patient. The three-step analysis approach gives observable, concrete values to esoteric perceptions and expectations. These values constitute a common esthetic language.

The consultation appointment should include a discussion of your

Are You a Candidate for Cosmetic Dentistry?*

Why change your smile? If you're happy with it, don't! But ask yourself the following questions:

Yes	No	
❑	❑	1. Are you self-confident about smiling?
❑	❑	2. Do you ever put your hand over your mouth when you smile?
❑	❑	3. Do you photograph better from one side of your face?
❑	❑	4. Is there someone you believe has a better smile than you?
❑	❑	5. Do you look at magazines and wish you had a smile as pretty as the models'?
❑	❑	6. When you read a fashion magazine, are your eyes drawn to the model's smile?
❑	❑	7. When you look at your smile in the mirror, do you see any defects in your teeth or gums?
❑	❑	8. Do you wish your teeth were whiter?
❑	❑	9. Are you satisfied with the way your gums look?
❑	❑	10. Do you show too many or too few teeth when you smile?
❑	❑	11. Do you show too much or too little gum when you smile?
❑	❑	12. Are your teeth too long or too short?
❑	❑	13. Are your teeth too wide or too narrow?
❑	❑	14. Are your teeth too square or too round?
❑	❑	15. Do you like the way your teeth are shaped?

If you answered "no" to every question except 1, 9, and 15, you are content with your smile.

Form 7-1

* From Goldstein RE. *Change Your Smile.* Chicago: Quintessence, 1997.

patient's perceived esthetic concerns. An esthetic self-evaluation combined with an in-office esthetic evaluation will provide much of the necessary information that can lead to a successful result. When your patients fill out a short evaluation form (Form 7-1), you are asking them to critically analyze their smile. This analysis may disclose aspects of themselves that they had never noticed, which creates an opportunity for you to actively discuss your patient's esthetic concerns and evaluate whether imaging will help in the communication process.

Many esthetic checklists are available for patient analysis.[2,3,4] No matter which form you choose, use it! In-depth forms help you to document the qualities of the patient's smile in detail. This analysis helps in your diagnosis, treatment planning, and laboratory communication.

Step 1: Esthetic Evaluation Form

To identify problems, a comprehensive diagnostic form is used. The importance of this form cannot be overemphasized; even if you have a certain idea in mind about the best way to proceed, the use of this form will either reinforce these ideas or inform you that the patient's expectations differ from your assumptions.[5]

The doctor and appropriate members of the dental team go through a series of open-ended questions, which are designed *not* to provoke a "yes" or "no" response. A key principle in this process lies in overcoming the patient's resistance to being told what to do and how to do it. People will support most those ideas they consider their own. You must therefore ask effective questions, listen carefully, and respond to the patient's answers. The most effective questions are open-ended, encouraging patients to express themselves. A close-ended question, which produces a "yes" or "no" response, discourages patients from thinking and talking and ultimately elicits limited information.

Examples of effective questions are found on the evaluation form (Form 7-2). The use of this form not only provides the information necessary for esthetic evaluation, but encourages involvement by the patient's family and friends as well as members of the treatment team. It serves to further strengthen trust amongst all parties. The patient will feel that his or her needs and desires are considered important and encourage discussion on specific concerns. Effective questions focus on the subjective needs of the patient. The simple question, "If there was anything you could change about your smile, what would it be?" serves to open up communication and to allow the patient to speak of any dissatisfaction with his or her present smile. The form then asks whether the patient is attracted to natural-looking teeth, or the perfectly straight, white, media-image look. The answers will guide you toward an effective solution based on patient expectations, while revealing any unrealistic expectations. You then have the opportunity for discussion and resolution before—not during or after—treatment.

*Esthetic Evaluation**

Patient ______________________ Examiner ______________________ Date ____ /____/ ____

1. Effective Questions

A. If there was anything you could change about your smile, what would it be?

____

____

____

B. Do you like the media image of perfectly straight, white teeth, or are you content with healthy, clean, natural-looking teeth?

❑ Media image ❑ Natural looking

C. History of esthetic change ____

____

____

____

D. Previous records

Do you have any previous photographs of your smile to aid in your esthetic treatment planning?

❑ Yes ❑ No

2. Facial Analysis

A. Full smile

1. Interpupillary line to occlusal plane
   ❑ Parallel ❑ Canted right ❑ Canted left
2. Midline relationship of teeth (central incisor) to face (philtrum)
   ❑ Symmetric ❑ Right of center ❑ Left of center
3. Relationship of lips to face (lip symmetry)
   ❑ Symmetric ❑ Right ❑ Left

B. Lips at rest

1. Upper lip
   ❑ Full ❑ Average ❑ Thin
2. Lower lip
   ❑ Full ❑ Average ❑ Thin
3. Lips
   ❑ Prominent ❑ Retruded
4. Tooth exposure at rest
   Upper _________ mm Lower _________ mm

C. Profile

1. Nasolabial angle
   ❑ Normal approximately 90° ❑ Prominant maxilla < 90° ❑ Retruded maxilla > 90°
2. Rickets E-Plane
   Draw from tip of nose to chin.
   Measure upper lip to E-plane and lower lip to E-plane.
   – upper lip 4 mm to E-plane
   – lower lip 2 mm to E-plane
   ❑ Within normal ❑ Convex ❑ Concave

Nasolabial Edge

Rickets E-Plane

If maxilla is prominent, nasolabial angle is < 90˚, or profile is convex . . . consider smaller, less dominant maxillary anterior restorations.

If maxilla is retruded, nasolabial angle is > 90˚, or profile is concave . . . consider more dominant, labially placed maxillary anterior restorations.

Form 7-2

3. Dentofacial Analysis

A. Upper lip

❑ Average ❑ High 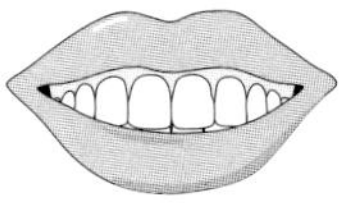 ❑ Low

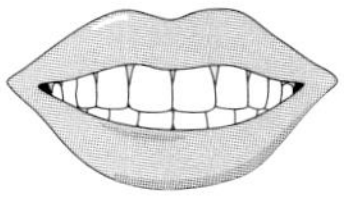

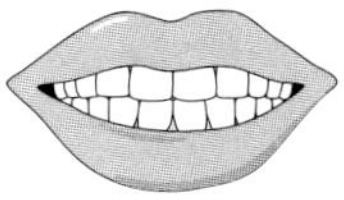

B. Incisal edge to lower lip

❑ Convex curve ❑ Straight 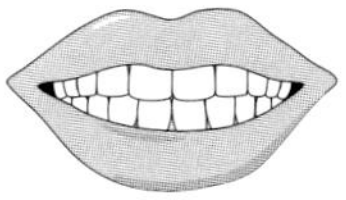 ❑ Reverse

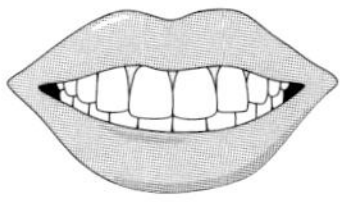

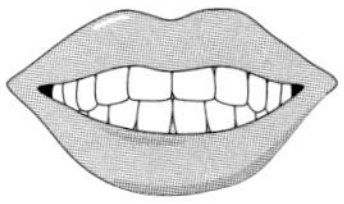

C. Tooth–Lower lip position

❑ Touching ❑ Not touching 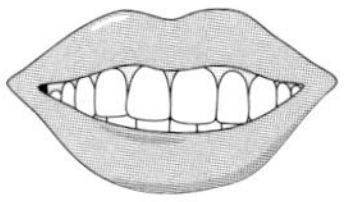 ❑ Slightly covered

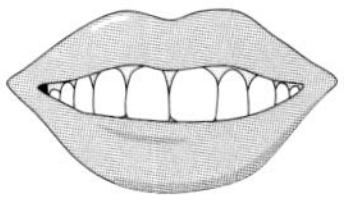

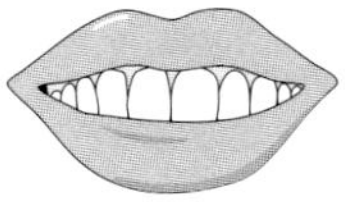

D. Full smile . . . number of teeth exposed

❑ 6 ❑ 8 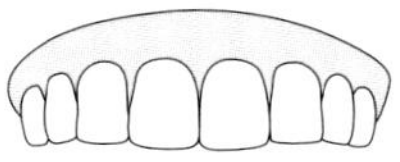 ❑ 10 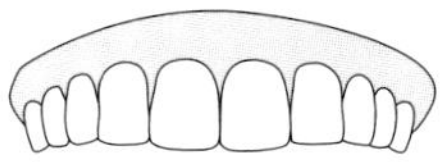 ❑ 16

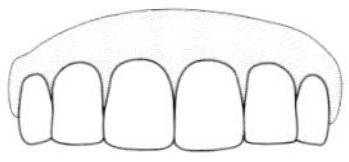

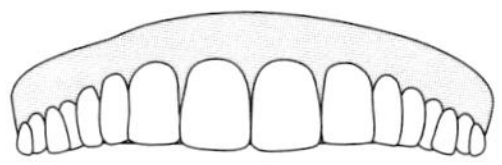

E. Midline . . . relationship of central incisors to philtrum

❑ Center ❑ Right of center 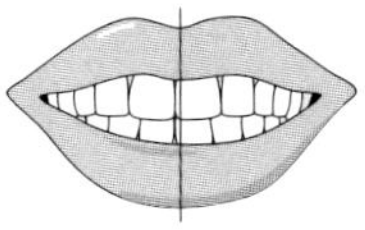 ❑ Left of center

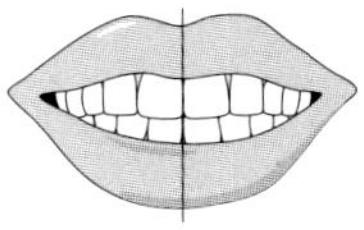

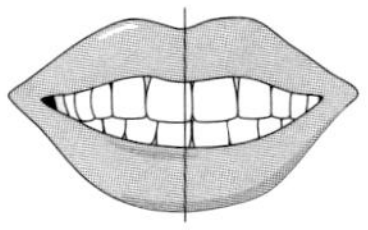

F. Midline . . . skewing to left or right

❑ Right ❑ Left 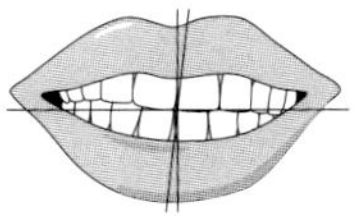 ❑ Straight

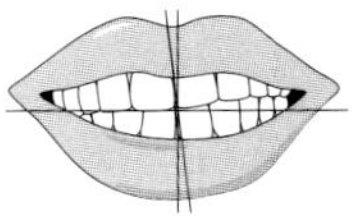

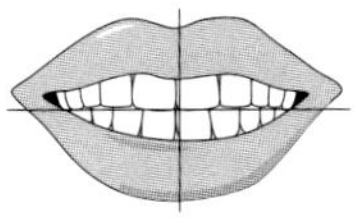

G. Bilateral negative space

❑ Normal ❑ Increased

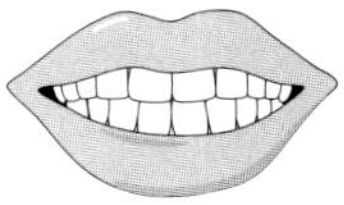

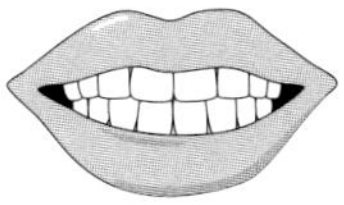

H. Phonetics

1. F-V sounds . . . incisal edge of maxillary centrals on wet/dry line of lower lip ❑ Yes ❑ No
2. S sound . . . closest speaking space—clear sound ❑ Yes ❑ No

4. Dental Analysis

A. Proportion of central incisors

Measure with calipers

Height

Width

Width:Height (W:H) Ratio ❑ > 80% ❑ < 80%

(The ideal width is 80% of the height)

B. Proportion of central to lateral to canine

Measure with calipers

.6 1 1.6

central width ________ mm

lateral width ________ mm

cuspid width ________ mm

C. Axial inclinations

Draw in misalignment

D. Gingival and tooth characteristics

Draw in clinical height of gingiva

❑ Gingival asymmetry

❑ Mucogingival problem

5. Diagnostic Information

1. Gingival height asymmetry ❑ Yes ❑ No
   location ________
2. Dark triangles ❑ Yes ❑ No
   location ________
3. Discolored gingiva ❑ Yes ❑ No
   location ________
4. Overcontoured crowns ❑ Yes ❑ No
   location ________
5. Poor crown margins (open) ❑ Yes ❑ No
   location ________
6. Active periodontal problems (probings) ❑ Yes ❑ No
   location ________
7. Mobility and/or furcation ❑ Yes ❑ No
   location ________
8. Endodontic lesion ❑ Yes ❑ No
   location ________
9. Occlusion—wear facets/incisal wear ❑ Yes ❑ No
   location ________
10. Continuous progression from canine distally (coincidence of curves) ❑ Yes ❑ No
    location ________
11. Flared teeth ❑ Yes ❑ No
    location ________
12. Diastema ❑ Yes ❑ No
    location ________
13. Overlapped teeth ❑ Yes ❑ No
    location ________
14. Chipped teeth ❑ Yes ❑ No
    location ________
15. Discolored teeth ❑ Yes ❑ No
    location ________
16. Surface texture . . . smooth ❑ Yes ❑ No
    ❑ Light ❑ Medium ❑ High

6. Diagnostic Information Checklist

❑ Esthetic evaluation form ❑ Study casts . . . diagnostic wax-ups ❑ Computer imaging or similar visualization tool

7. Additional Notes ________

The dental team follows three stages of analysis, according to a concept developed by Leonard Abrams. This involves starting with the full face and zooming in closer for an evaluation of the teeth.

- Facial (Fig 7-1)
- Dentofacial (lips, gingiva, and teeth) (Fig 7-2)
- Dental (teeth and gingiva) (Fig 7-3)

Facial symmetry, lip symmetry, smile line, horizontal and vertical tooth display, midline, and tooth contour are reviewed in a checklist style. A member of the dental team should refer to each specific point and note the condition. The process is similar to a camera zooming in on a subject, beginning with the whole face and then focusing on the teeth and reviewing the significant elements along the way. An assistant may be used to call out the basic element, with the dentist providing the evaluation (eg, Assistant: "Lipline: high, medium, low." Doctor: "low"). The assistant checks the finding on the form. The esthetic evaluation form may then serve as an information source for computer imaging.

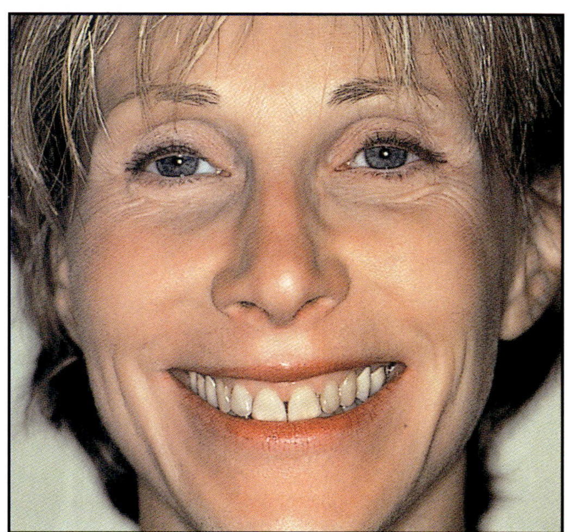

Fig 7-1 *Evaluate the face as a whole.*

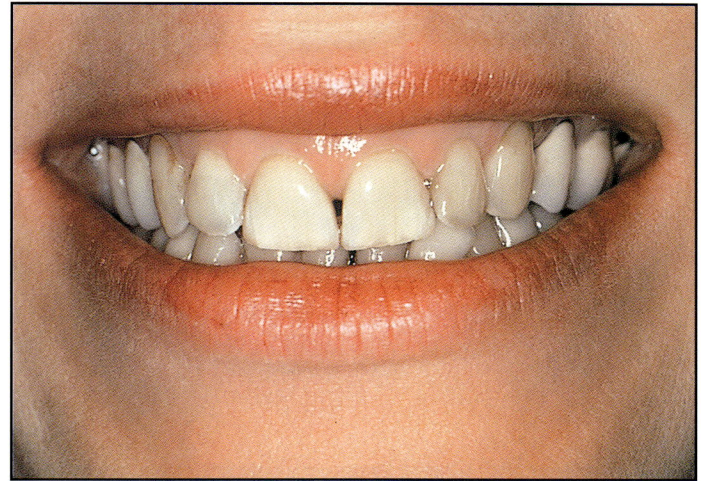

Fig 7-2 *"Zoom in" to analyze how the lips, gingiva, and teeth form the oral apparatus.*

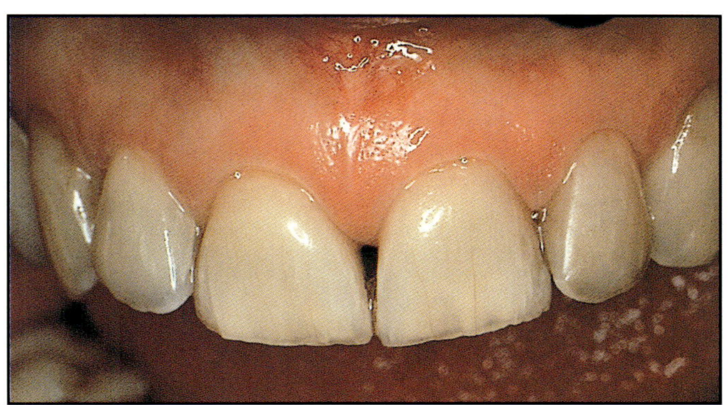

Fig 7-3 *Finally, concentrate on the relationship between the gingiva and the teeth.*

Step 2: Computer Imaging

This task is again a combined effort of the dental team. The assistant/technician should be able to take the picture, put the image in the proper file, and initiate the imaging. The procedure is a critical learning experience wherein the dentist and his or her team bring their knowledge of esthetics to bear and, more important, involve the patient in the identification of the problems and the visualization of solutions.

It is important for the dental team to establish rapport with the patient and become effective listeners.

The patient is seated in front of the screen, and a professional-quality "before" picture is taken with proper lighting, angulation, and camera distance. Leading questions have already been asked of the patient from a clear, structured checklist of the important elements of the smile. Any possible asymmetries, rotations, "dark triangle areas," etc, have been delineated; you now have a good overall understanding of the patient's situation and needs. At this point, imaging allows for these problems and projected corrections to be observed and manipulated during a discussion with the patient, ensuring that his or her perspective is taken into account.

Two images will be produced: one that is unaltered, and one that will show the proposed changes (Fig 7-4). The patient can make specific requests as to whether a gap can be closed, if teeth can be made lighter, or if the show of gingiva can be reduced. As the dialogue proceeds, the changes are made on the proposed image side of the screen. It is important for the dental team to establish rapport with the patient and become effective listeners. They should speak as little as possible and only to coax information from the patient or to clarify a technical issue. This type of communication will continue to reinforce the high-trust relationship necessary between you and the patient.

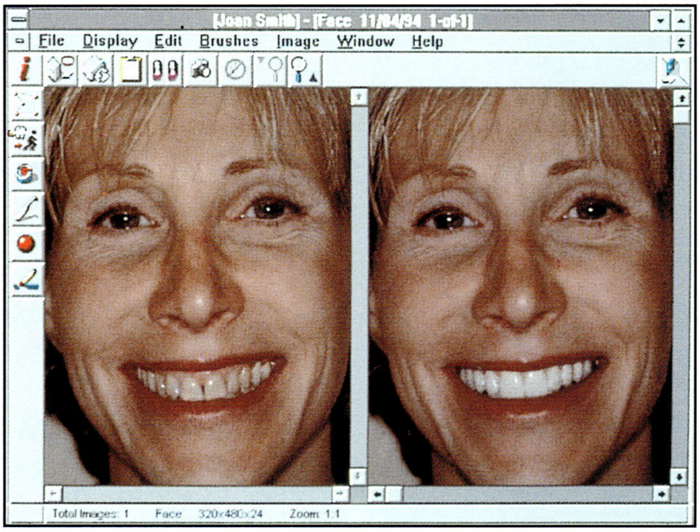

Fig 7-4 *The computer image is finalized using the data accumulated from the esthetic evaluation form (Form 7-2).*

Step 3: Diagnostic Wax-Up

After a study cast is made (Fig 7-5), a diagnostic wax-up may be made (Fig 7-6) to verify the proposed changes from the computer imaging session. This is an important part of the three-step analysis, serving to verify that what was projected with the two-dimensional computer image can actually be achieved. Without this step, the computer image may often be misleading to both patient and clinician. Some basic rules for the diagnostic wax-up are based on the fundamentals of esthetics:

1. Starting with the central incisors, develop either dominance (a width-to-height ratio of 80%) or divine proportion at a ratio of 1.6:1. You must give information to the technician concerning the tooth length (final incisal edge length for the wax-up) as determined by the esthetic evaluation form and the computer image.
2. Seek symmetry at the midline, gingiva (all aspects including height), and contours of the central incisors (ie, line angles mirror-imaging each other at the midline).
3. Use the law of golden proportion for proper tooth-to-tooth proportion. The ratio of widths of the central incisor, lateral incisor, and cuspid is 1.6 to 1.0.
4. Direct the axial inclination of the teeth toward the distal.
5. Make sure that the incisal embrasures become progressively larger as they move from the central incisor to the cuspid.
6. Insert proper line angles that are parallel to the long axis of the tooth.
7. Use tooth texture and incisal edge contour to help create a natural and younger look.
8. Properly position the gingival height; either remove or add pink wax to simulate proposed gingival changes. View the tissue height and relate it to the length of the tooth.

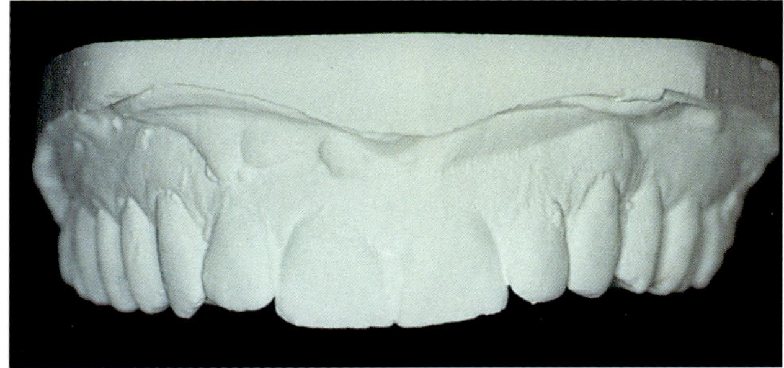

Fig 7-5 The study cast.

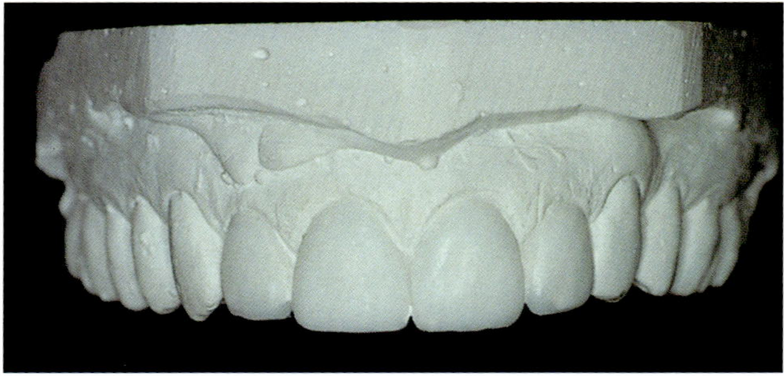

Fig 7-6 The diagnostic wax-up is made to verify that the esthetic enhancements in the two-dimensional computer image can actually be accomplished.

In summary, the esthetic evaluation form is used to collect the information necessary to evaluate the smile, face, teeth, gingiva, and phonetics in a checklist fashion. The use of effective questioning and equally attentive listening skills is essential. The computer image continues the evaluation process and the search for solutions. As interaction develops between the parties, necessary changes are identified and the solutions are visualized. The diagnostic wax-up verifies the workability of the two-dimensional images generated by the computer.

Completing these three steps generates significant insights that contribute to the success of the esthetic treatment. When the dental team and the patient work together, communication is maximized, and a clear understanding of the patient's perception of esthetics is reached. Effective questions help build strong relationships between the patient and the dental team, allowing the patient to drive the decision-making process in the esthetic diagnosis. The three-step analysis serves to increase the probability of successful and consistent treatment, while improving both your own and your team's general understanding of esthetic concepts. Once the problem is identified and the solution is visualized, choosing the appropriate technique is easier (Figs 7-7 to 7-13).

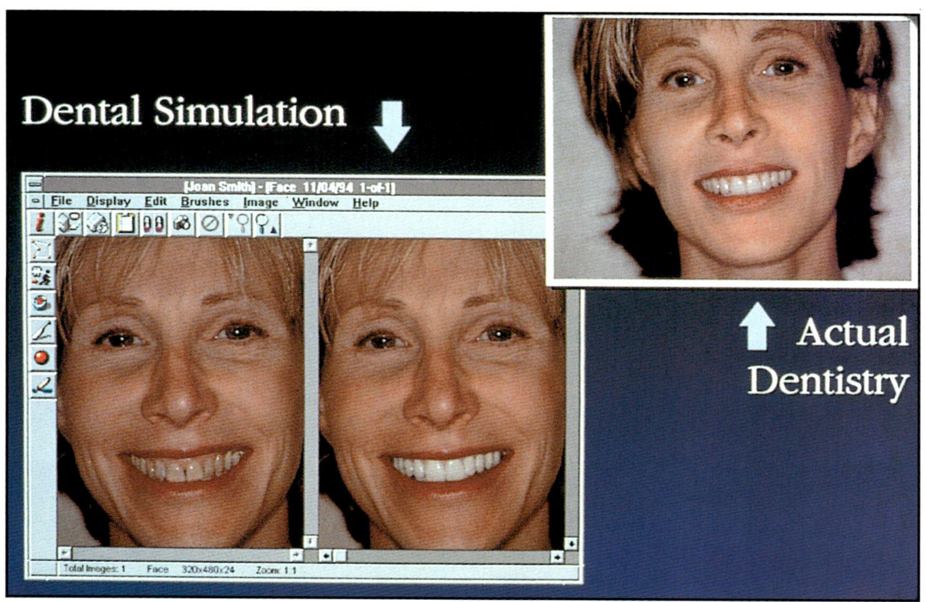

Fig 7-7 Note the close approximation of the computer image to the actual dental treatment.

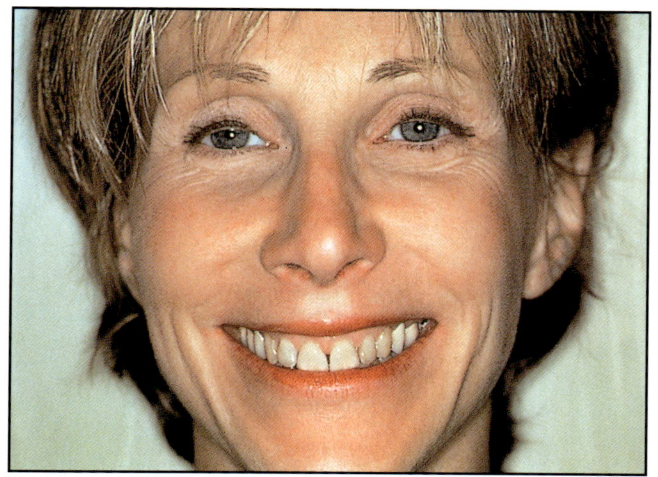

Fig 7-8 Full face before.

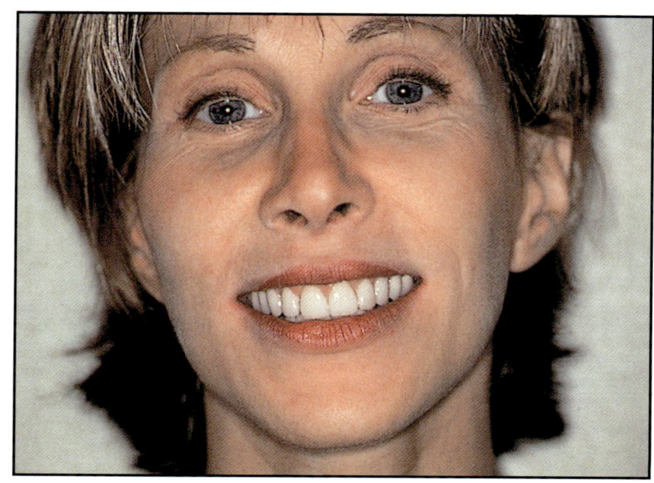

Fig 7-9 Full face after.

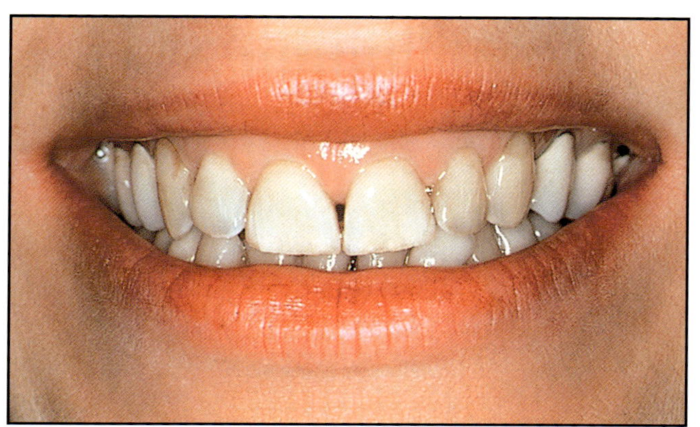

Fig 7-10 Smile before.

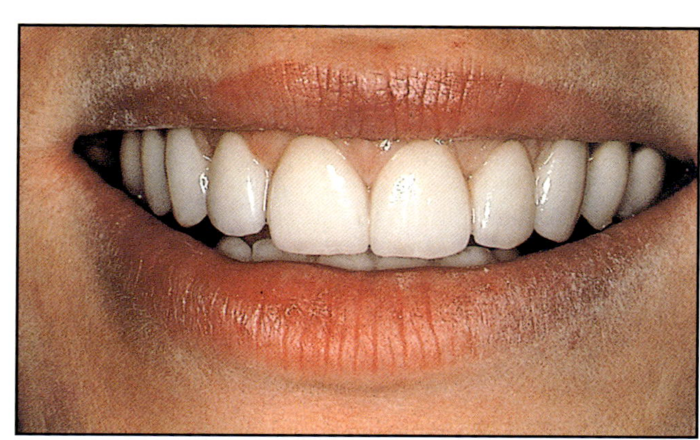

Fig 7-11 Smile after.

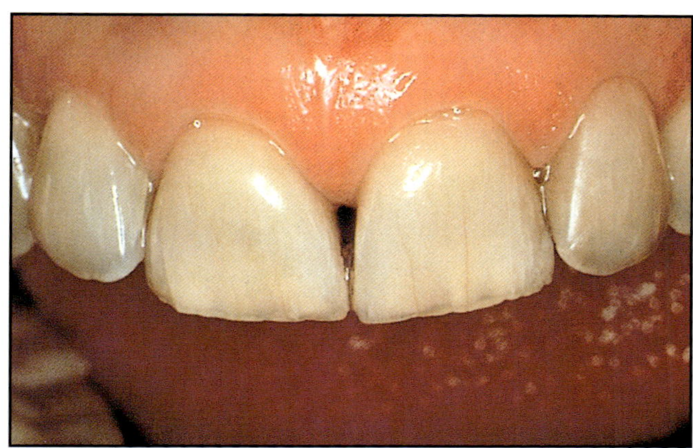

Fig 7-12 Close-up before.

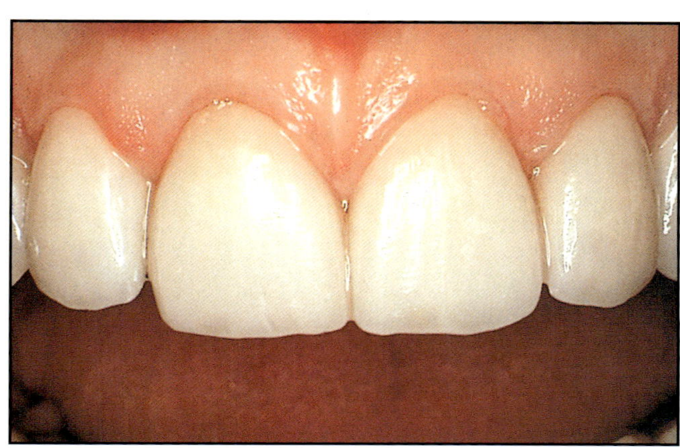

Fig 7-13 Close-up after.

References

1. Gane D, Levine JB. Imaging the esthetic case: A structured 3-step analysis. Esthetic Dentistry Update 1995;6:85–90.
2. Levine JB. Esthetic Diagnosis. London: Current Science, 1995;9–17.
3. Dawson PF. Evaluation, Diagnosis, and Treatment of Occlusal Problems. St. Louis: Mosby, 1995.
4. Goldstein RE. Esthetics in Dentistry. Toronto: BC Decker, 1998.
5. Brisman AS. Esthetics. A comparison of dentists' and patients' concepts. JADA 1980:100;345.

Computer *Techniques* to Design a Smile

8

David Gane, DDS, BSc, and Barbara Wagner, RDH

Computer images acquired for simulation purposes form an integral part of the patient record. When used in combination with the study casts and radiographs, these images are invaluable tools for diagnosis, treatment planning, and case presentation. In this chapter, you will find specific suggestions on how to use computer imaging technology to help patients and others visualize the esthetic potential of various procedures in addition to aiding diagnosis and treatment planning.

Esthetic Evaluation

After the acquisition of the appropriate facial, dentofacial, and dental images, the esthetic evaluation begins by prompting the patient with a series of open-ended questions designed to reveal what the patient would like to change about his or her smile (see the esthetic evaluation form, Chapter 7). Such an approach encourages patients to express their wants with respect to treatment. Next, a careful analysis of the facial, dentofacial, and dentoalveolar views is then performed. Facial symmetry, lip symmetry, smile line, horizontal and vertical tooth display, midline, and tooth contour are reviewed in an orderly fashion. This information checklist facilitates the clear identification of existing esthetic problems while taking into account the patient's treatment expectations. The checklist then becomes the design blueprint for the cosmetic image simulations.[1,2]

Golden Proportion and Computer Imaging

Computers are giving new meaning to the term *diagnosis* in restorative dentistry. Your ability to successfully predict results can improve when computer imaging is used to determine the ideal tooth position as well as tooth form and size. Actual tooth measurements derived from the imaging session produce more accurate instructions for referral sources or the laboratory.

One of the best ways computer imaging can aid the restorative dentist in determining tooth size is by incorporating the "golden" or "divine" proportion concept into arch and tooth evaluation. This ancient theory states that for objects to be in esthetic harmony, they should exist in the ratio of .618 to 1[3,4] (Fig 8-1). In dentistry, certain groups of teeth are theoretically proportionate to each other in this ratio. According to Levin[5] "the [perceived] width of the [maxillary] central incisor is in golden proportion to the width of the lateral incisor." Similarly, "the width of the [maxillary] lateral incisor is in golden proportion to the width of the canine." Research by Preston[6] states that these proportions are derived from the *apparent* size of the teeth as viewed directly from the anterior aspect. Preston concludes that "although the advocated ratios may provide a result that is esthetically pleasing, they are not the ratios found in nature." For many patients, this theory and the ratio of the golden proportion can be quite useful, especially as a starting point in achieving a harmonious and esthetic anterior segment.

In calculating the most esthetic arrangement of the maxillary arch from the labial approach, it is essential to understand that the golden proportion works in two dimensions rather than three. In other words, it is important to look at the arch in a smiling or retracted frontal view when applying the golden proportion: even though the arch curves posteriorly, the actual tooth width is not as important as is the amount of tooth exposed to the frontal view (Fig 8-2a and b). It can also be helpful, in esthetic consultation with your patients, to explain the golden proportion. Show them how their own proportions differ from the proposed ideal, and show how their appearance would change if the proportions were brought into harmony (Fig 8-3). This can foster a better understanding of the problem as well as the solution.

Some imaging programs incorporate the golden proportion directly into the application toolbar; others can be programmed to use it. The computer can then use a known measurement to extrapolate the proper proportion for an esthetic restoration.

When you include this simple mathematical equation in your computer analysis, you make it easier to diagnose various esthetic problems and arrive at the best solution.

Fig 8-1 The ancient theory of golden proportion states that for objects to be in esthetic harmony, they should exist in the ratio of 1 to .618 or 1.618 to 1. In dentistry, teeth and groups of teeth are theoretically proportionate to each other in this ratio.

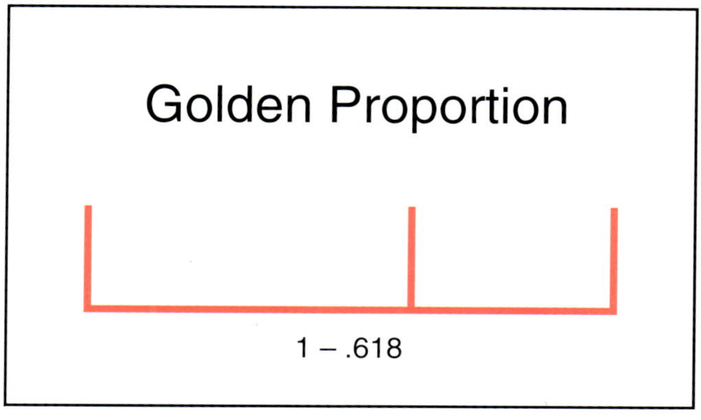

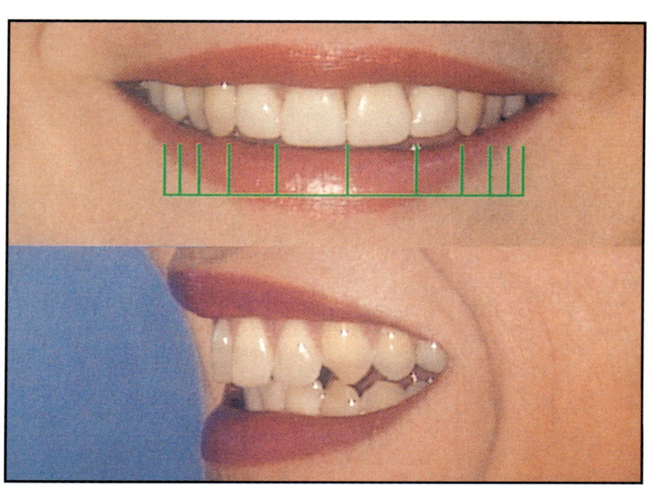

Fig 8-2a The golden proportion concept is derived from the apparent size of the teeth as viewed directly from the anterior aspect. The actual tooth width is not as important as is the amount of tooth exposed to the frontal view. It is essential to understand that the golden proportion works in two dimensions, not three.

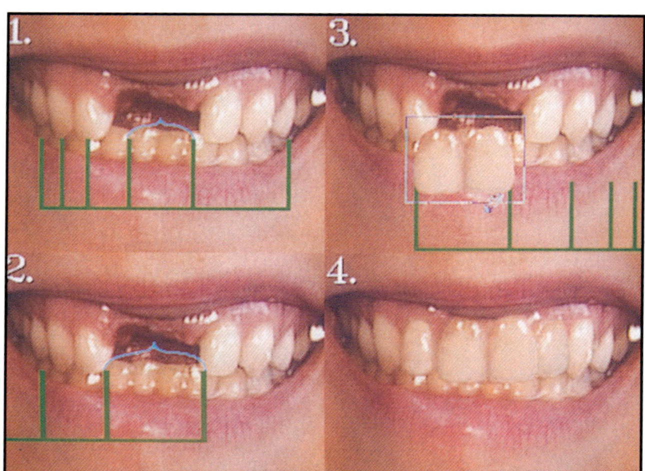

Fig 8-2b The golden proportion is used to select appropriately proportioned incisors for this partially edentulous patient.

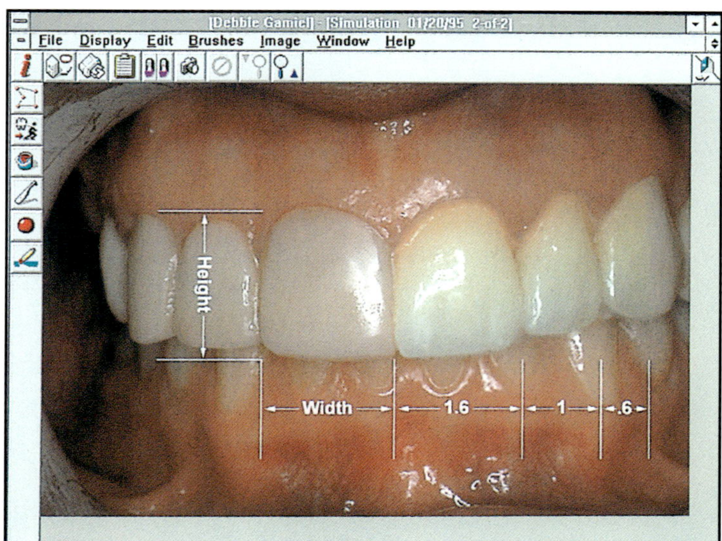

Fig 8-3 During esthetic consultation, explain the golden proportion to the patient and how his or her own proportions differ from the proposed ideal.

Software Tools to Plan a New Smile

The following will acquaint you with the basic tools commonly available in computer imaging systems. Specific examples of how to use these tools in a variety of clinical applications are offered. Of necessity, this discussion is general and does not cover the specifics of every available system.

Move, Framed Move, and Cut and Paste

Suppose a patient presents with a badly chipped, stained, or nonvital left central incisor, but has an attractive right central incisor. The ideal solution would be to outline the attractive tooth, reverse it, and position it over the unattractive contralateral tooth. That is a typical application of the *move* function, which lets you define a portion of the image and reposition it elsewhere in the image (Fig 8-4). The designated portion can be enlarged or reduced proportionately or disproportionately, flipped over, turned upside down, or rotated. The move function is important because it allows you to use sections of a natural tooth, preserving all of its variants of color, texture, and shape. With less sophisticated systems, you must draw tooth shapes with a solid color, which gives a flat, unnatural appearance.

Draw

The draw function allows you to draw with a solid color on the screen (also called the *canvas*). This is useful to simulate repairs of small chips and defects (Fig 8-5) but should not be used for larger restorations. Teeth are complex variations of colors; using the draw function too extensively will give the image a "paint by number" look.

Copy, Duplicate

This feature copies a defined part of the image to another place on the screen. For example, to show full-mouth reconstruction or dentures, you might "borrow" a set of teeth from a tooth bank—a computerized library stocked with images of teeth. However, these ideal teeth probably will not fit the patient's smile line exactly. The copy function lets you duplicate the lips from the "before" image on the "after" image, thus restoring the natural lip line relationships over the new teeth (Fig 8-6).

Wash or Tint

This function goes by different names, but, in general, it means overlaying color to the image without obscuring the original color and texture beneath. This is most commonly used for bleaching simulations (Fig 8-7), but it can also be useful for taking the red, puffy look out of diseased gingival tissue by placing a faint tint of white over the dark red. Conversely, you can simulate the early stages of periodontitis by applying a dark-red tint on an image of normal tissue. Other uses include color characterization, such as using a medium-gray tint to simulate incisal translucency or a mid-range yellow to show coronal highlights.

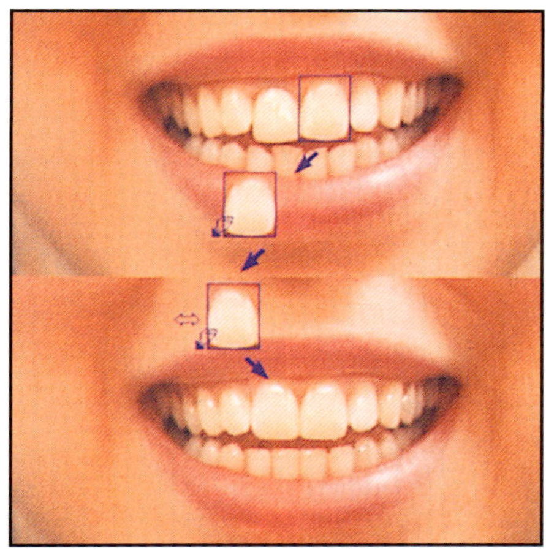

Fig 8-4 *To correct the tooth size relationship and tooth-to-tissue ratio, the desirable tooth is framed, flipped over, and "moved" or "cut-and-pasted" into the proper position.*

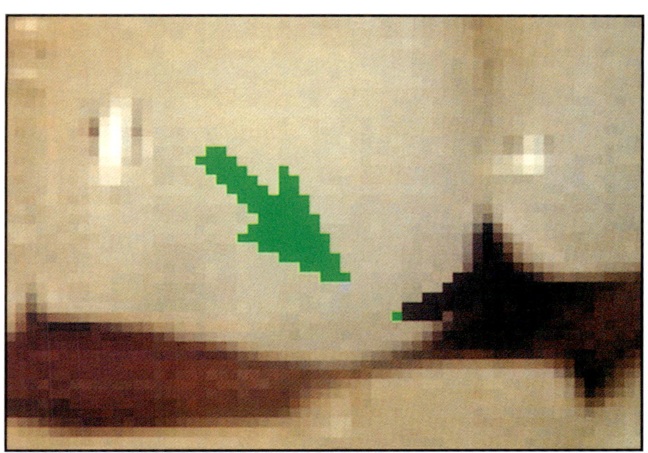

Fig 8-5 *The distal aspect of this incisor needs reshaping. The dark background color is "drawn" over the tooth area to be contoured.*

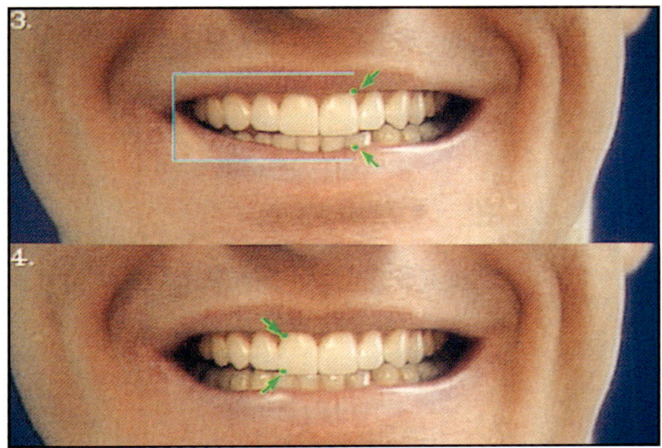

Fig 8-6 *A new set of teeth is selected from a tooth bank and placed over this man's smile. Notice the patient's original lip corner at the left side of the framed move. The lips from the framed move are being erased and the patient's old lips "copied" back onto the face.*

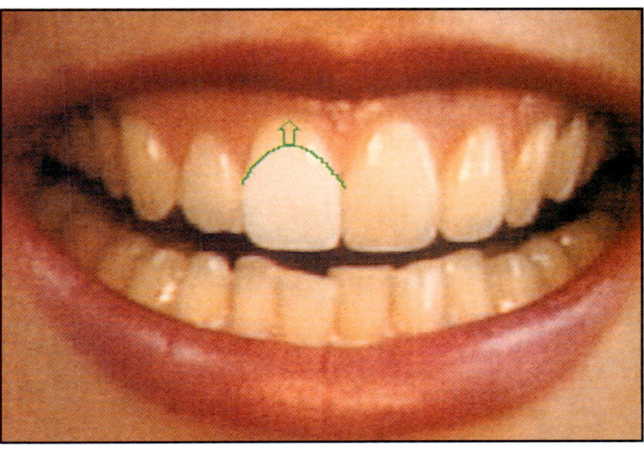

Fig 8-7 *Lightening of this tooth is achieved by placing a "wash" or "tint" of color over its surface. Notice how the incisal area retains its subtle hue variation and the facial highlights are maintained. (If this lightening were done with the "draw" mode, the result would eliminate the incisal translucency and the light reflections.)*

Erase

Since imaging systems typically can keep a copy of the original image in the background, this tool enables you to restore portions of the image to its original state (Fig 8-8).

Undo

This function restores the entire image to its unaltered state, undoing all the modifications you have made (Fig 8-9). It can also be used to reverse only the last procedure. This valuable feature is not available on all systems.

Blend or Smooth

Once you have finished modifying an image, this function averages the color of the pixels to eliminate the sharp edit line areas (Fig 8-10). An intensity scale adjusts from slight to maximum blend. Blend should be used sparingly since it may soften detail that you want to make obvious to the patient or the laboratory.

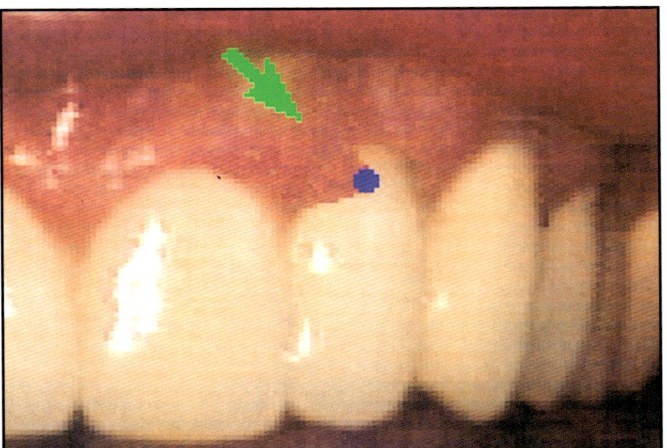

Fig 8-8 The original tissue contours of this lateral incisor are brought back by "erasing" or covering the new tooth. The blue dot is drawn only over the areas to be covered with the patient's original tissue height.

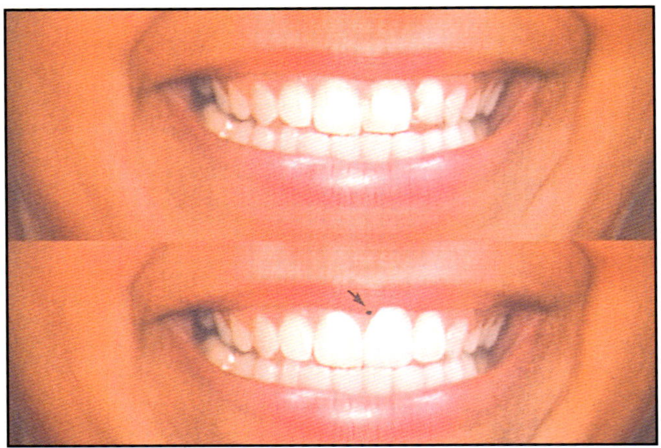

Fig 8-9 Similar to the erase feature, the undo feature restores all or part of an image to its original state.

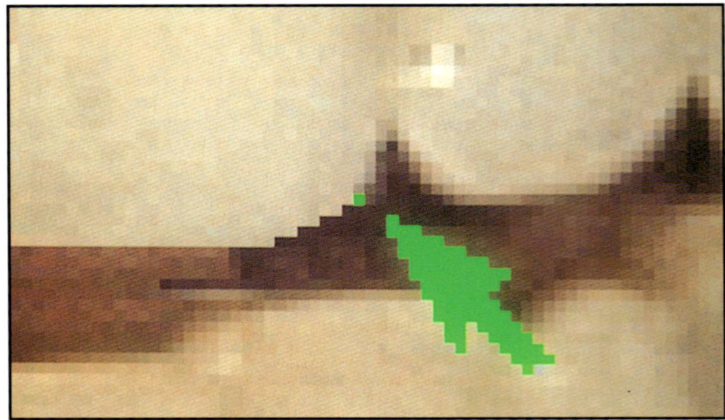

Fig 8-10 When functions such as a framed move or draw are used, the computer leaves sharp or jagged lines. These lines must be smoothed to make the image appear natural. Enlarging the area to be blended or smoothed will often enhance the result.

Clear

This function erases the current image from the screen.

Scale Set, Measurement, or Analyze

This function, which goes by several names, allows you to set a scale from a known measurement, such as the width of a tooth. Once the scale is set, the system can compute other measurements of the same image (Fig 8-11).

Pan or Zoom

This function provides a close-up view for detailed work by enlarging an image or a portion of it (Fig 8-12).

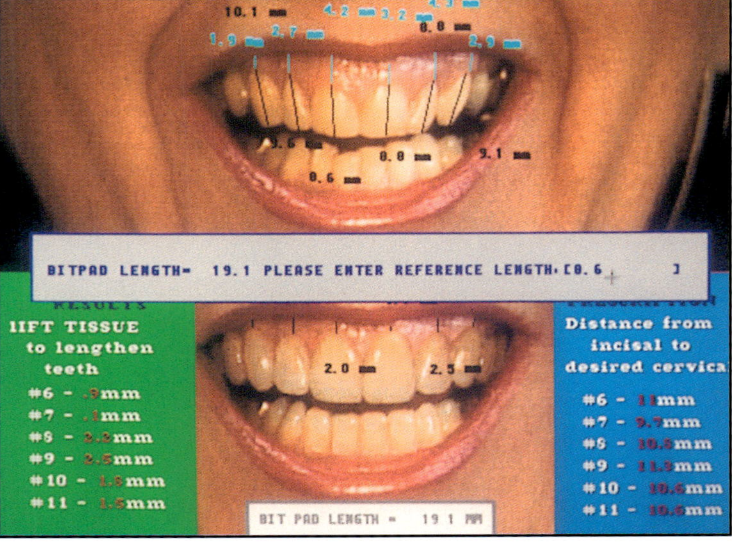

Fig 8-11 *A "periodontal prescription" is used to communicate the measurements needed of the teeth and tissue after surgical healing. Once one tooth length measurement is made, the computer interpolates the remaining tooth measurements using the same scale.*

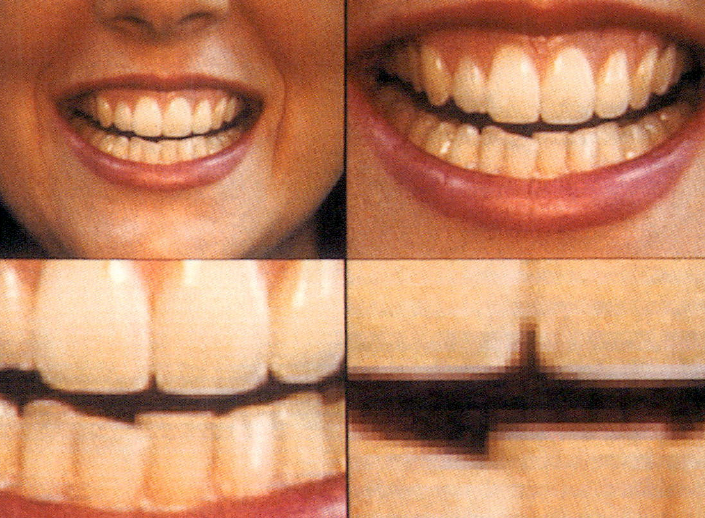

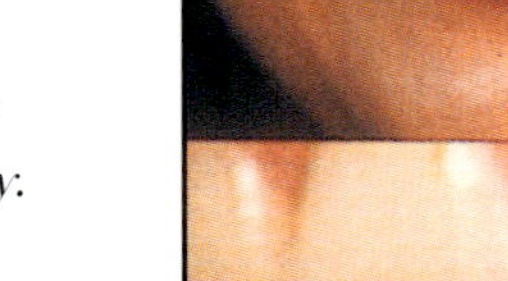

Fig 8-12 *The image viewed can be enlarged successively, usually with the touch of one key.*

Guidelines for computer simulations

- Work from an esthetic evaluation checklist that facilitates the clear identification of esthetic problems and considers the patient's desires and treatment expectations.
- Make the most conservative changes first to see if this will satisfy your patient's needs. If the patient is present during your imaging alterations, these changes should be imaged quickly to capture your patient's immediate interest. Tooth whitening, cosmetic contouring, and tooth replacement are examples of procedures that can be easily simulated in the presence of the patient.
- Enlarge the image to make changes, if necessary. Use the pan and zoom function for the finest detail possible.
- For the most life-like results, use the cut-and-paste mode, which allows you to copy and move teeth, or portions of teeth, from one place to another.
- Simulate natural color gradations by adding a little yellow or yellow-brown in the cervical third (Fig 8-13). Violet, light blue, or gray on the incisal edges can give the appearance of translucence.
- If the modified area is more sharply defined than the remainder of the image, blend to soften the edges. Keep incisal edges sharp and in focus.
- Step back occasionally for a better perspective of the image.

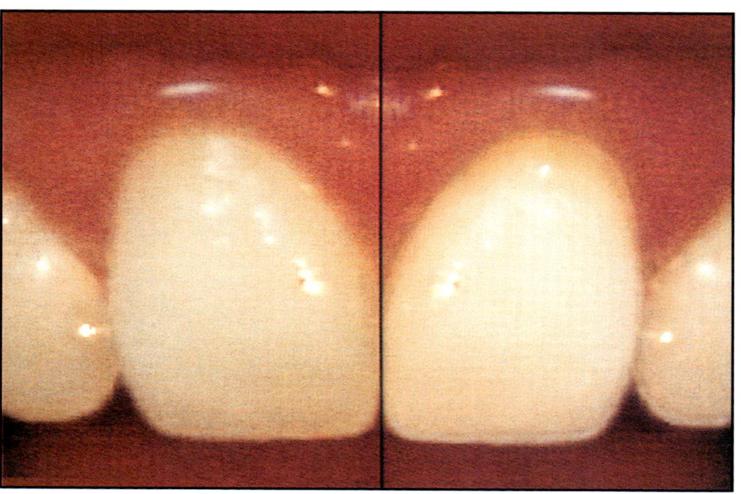

Fig 8-13 *An extra wash of color is added to the cervical aspect of the left central incisor and needs to be blended.*

Creating Windows and Banks

Most of us have had patients show a page from a magazine and say, "I wish my smile looked like this," or "This hairstyle is the one for me." With imaging technology, you can show patients precisely how they would look with that smile or hairstyle. These changes are particularly useful when the remedy for severe problems, such as staining or crowding, can be imaged more expediently by borrowing a new smile from another image.

Windows

Library images can be stored separately under their own file names on the computer (Fig 8-14). When recalled to the screen, windows can be sized and positioned as needed to fit into another image. Using windows, you can create your own computerized reference library of smiles or hairstyles for use during imaging consultations.

Often you will want to save only a portion of the image in a window. For example, suppose you want to add a hairstyle from a magazine photograph to your collection of hairstyles. You can retain the hairstyle of the model and eliminate the face and/or background:

1. Capture the image on screen with your input device.
2. "Paint out" with black the areas you do not need.
3. Save the window.
4. When the window is called back to the screen at a later time, the black areas will be transparent, and only the image of the hair will remain.

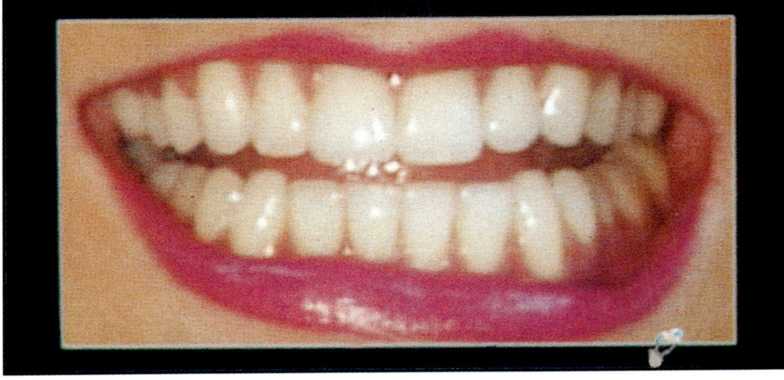

Fig 8-14 This smile is being saved as a window. At a later time, this smile or part of it may be chosen to replace part or all of another patient's smile.

Banks

A bank is a collection of many windows in a single image, enabling you to view them all at once (Fig 8-15). Hair banks and tooth banks can be purchased, or you can create your own.

To create a bank of windows:

1. Clear the screen.
2. One by one, load the windows that you have previously saved.
3. Shrink each to a size that preserves sufficient detail (Fig 8-16).
4. Arrange the windows on the screen.
5. Save the on-screen image as a bank (Fig 8-17).

For continuity, use the same background for all of your windows. Medium blue, gray, or black work best. Also, save hairstyles at the same set distance from the camera, so they will be the same size.

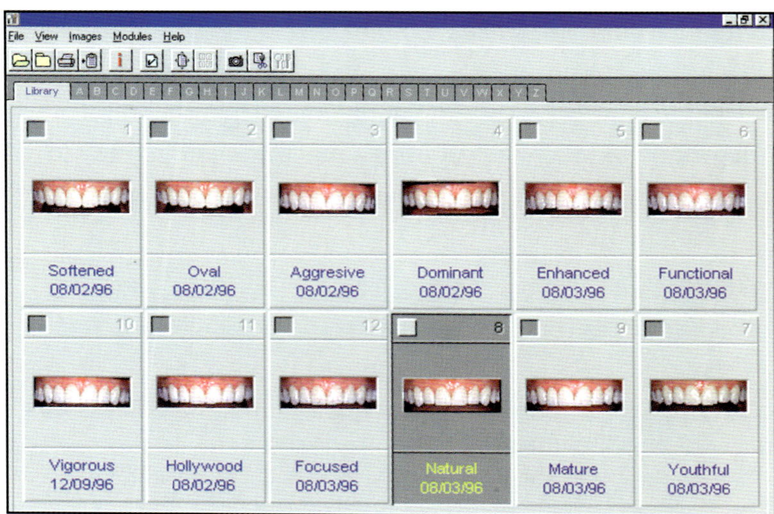

Fig 8-15a This library incorporates the twelve most common tooth arrangements and shapes. (Created by William G. Dickerson for Image FX Software Solutions Inc.)

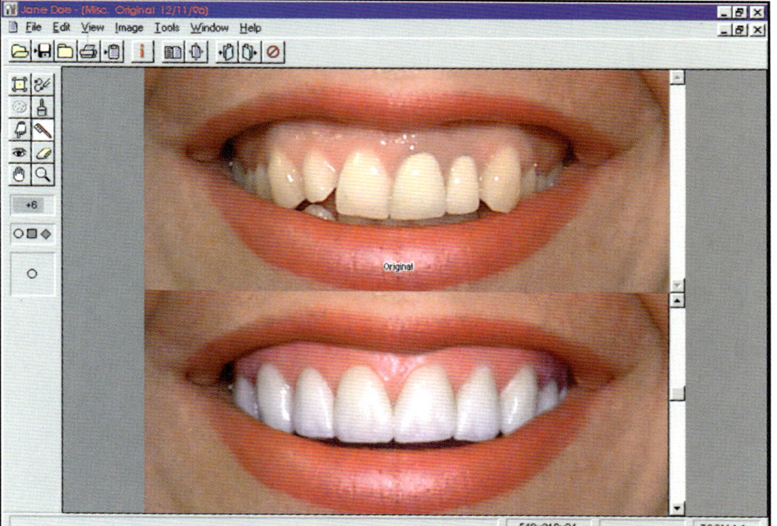

Fig 8-15b Selecting the appropriate library image and placing it within the patient's lips allows the patient and clinician to explore different esthetic treatment options.

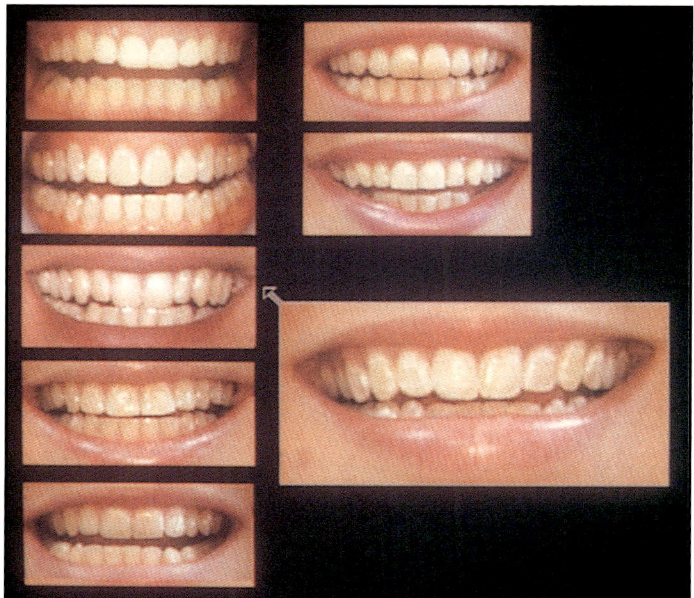

Fig 8-16 A smile bank is being created. The smiles are sized and arranged appropriately.

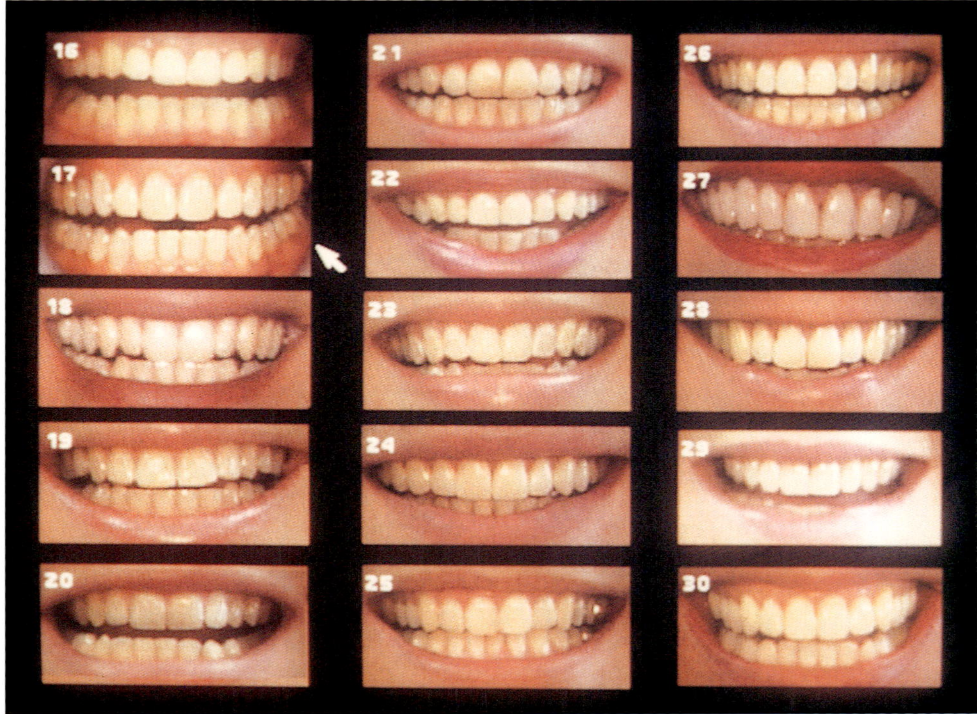

Fig 8-17 The completed bank of smiles is numbered for easy reference.

Using Teeth From the Tooth Bank

If you are completely changing a patient's teeth, it is relatively simple to replace them with a new set from a tooth bank.

1. Select the desired window from the tooth bank.
2. Position the new teeth over the teeth on the patient's "after" image (Fig 8-18a).
3. Position and size the teeth using the "before" image as a guide.
4. Use the erase or copy function to replace the lips over the teeth (Fig 8-18b).
5. Blend carefully and sparingly at minimum intensity.

If you plan to use a few teeth from the tooth bank and fit them into the patient's existing arch, you will probably have to adjust the color of the tooth-bank teeth:

1. Bring in the window from the tooth bank, as in Fig 8-18a.
2. Erase or copy all areas of the window you do not want and isolate the desired teeth.
3. Size and position the teeth properly on the patient's "after" image.
4. Save your changes.
5. If the new bank teeth are lighter than your patient's natural teeth:
   - Create a color spread between rust and brown (Fig 8-18c).
   - Tint the new teeth with about 20 percent of one of these colors (Fig 8-17d). (If the patient's original teeth are slightly reddish, for instance, choose a shade closer to the rust color.)
   - When you have the right shade overall, place a little extra wash color at the cervical aspect for a natural look.
6. Contour, blend, and replace the highlights (Fig 8-18e).

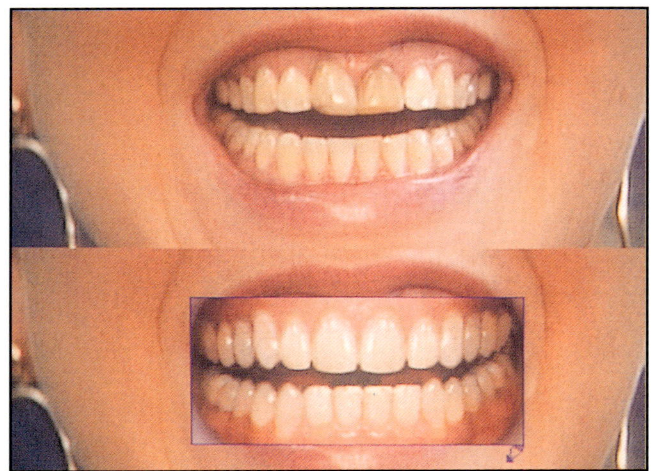

Fig 8-18a When significant changes are being made, teeth from the tooth bank are often needed. The number 17 smile from Fig 8-16 is chosen and placed over the patient's upper arch.

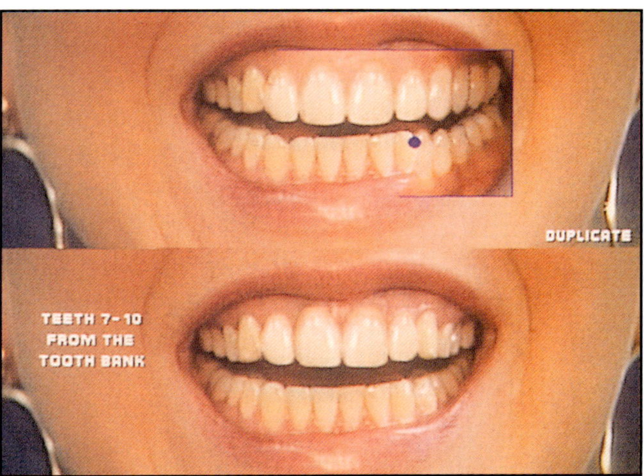

Fig 8-18b The patient's original tissues are now placed over the tooth-bank teeth.

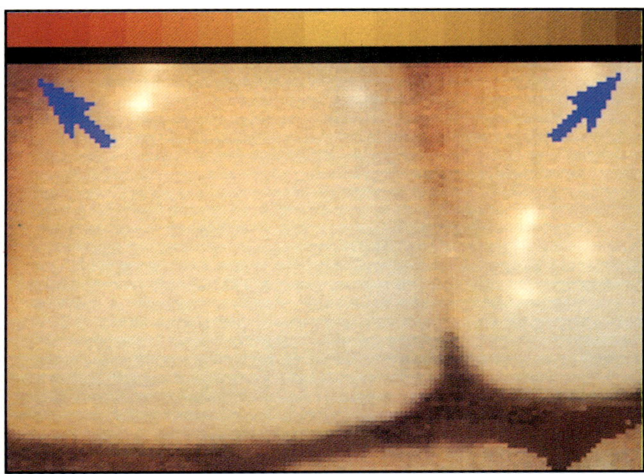

Fig 8-18c A color gradation may be used to achieve the proper hue.

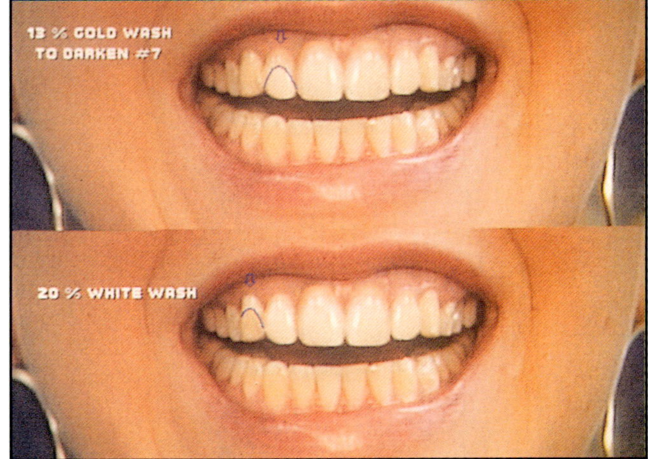

Fig 8-18d The color of the tooth-bank teeth may be adjusted as needed.

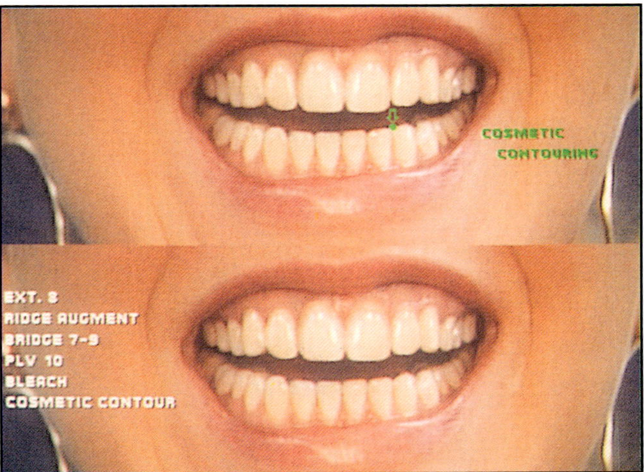

Fig 8-18e The completed image.

References

1. Levine JB. Esthetic diagnosis. Curr Opin Cosmet Dent 1995:9–17.
2. Gane D, Levine JB. Imaging the esthetic case: A structured three-step analysis. Esthetic Dentistry Update 1995;6:85–90.
3. Ricketts RE. The biologic significance of the divine proportion. Am J Orthod 1982; 81:351–370.
4. Ricketts RE. The divine proportion in facial esthetics. Clin Plast Surg 1982;9:401–422.
5. Levin EI. Dental Esthetics and the Golden Proportion. J Prosthet Dent 1978;40:244–252.
6. Preston J. The golden proportion revisited. J Esthet Dent 1993;5:247–251.

Designing a Smile

9

David Gane, DDS, BSc, and Barbara Wagner, RDH

Cosmetic Contouring

One of the simplest and most effective uses of computer imaging is illustrating the effects of cosmetic contouring—reshaping of the teeth to create an illusion of straightness.[1] Patients who are reluctant to have their teeth "ground away" can readily visualize the difference in before-and-after images and see how little tooth structure need be removed. This conservative and simple cosmetic procedure often can be imaged and performed in one visit.

Frontal full-face and close-up images of the smile work best to convey your ideas to the patient. A third, retracted close-up image may be needed when extensive crowding exists. Be sure to view your patient while he or she is standing as well as reclining, since crowded teeth generally look more severe from different vantage points. You may need to image and correct different views.

There are several ways to simulate cosmetic contouring with the computer. The most realistic effect can be achieved if you:

1. Frame and move sections of the existing teeth. This maintains natural-appearing light reflections and color.
2. Adjust the teeth for height and width.
3. Use the smallest stylus or brush tip to reshape the incisal edges.
4. Open incisal and gingival embrasures (Fig 9-1a and b).

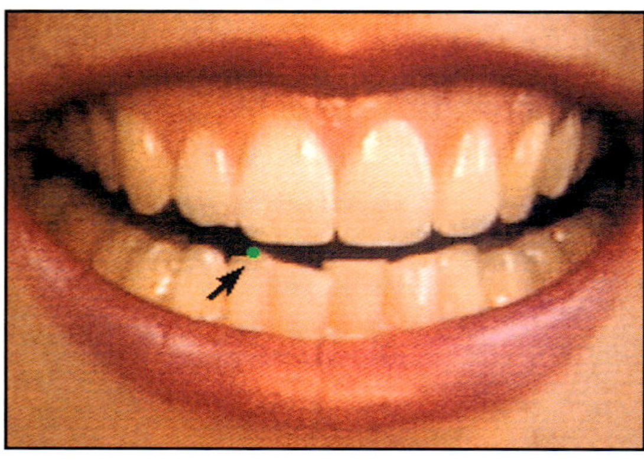

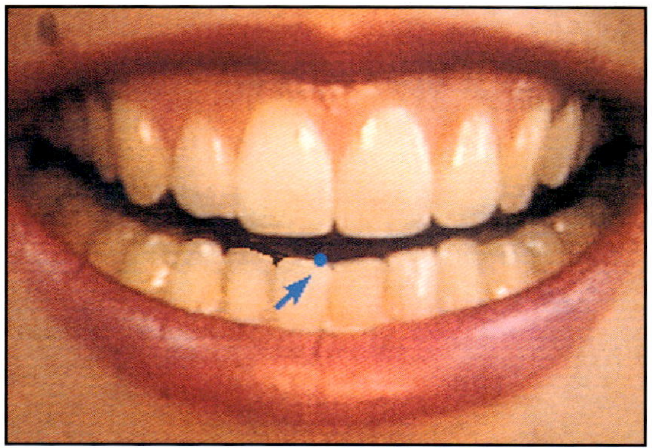

Fig 9-1a and b One of the simplest and most effective uses of computer imaging is to illustrate the effects of cosmetic contouring—reshaping of the teeth to create an illusion of straightness. Patients, who are often reluctant to have their teeth "ground away," can readily visualize the difference in before-and-after images and see how little tooth structure is actually removed. This inexpensive, cosmetic procedure often can be imaged and completed in one visit.

Many contouring changes can be imaged if you:

1. Magnify the image
2. Use a fine brush tip
3. "Pick up" the tongue color with the brush tip and use this color when making your corrections
4. Remove rough or irregular edges of the teeth
5. Define the embrasures

If the body of the tooth needs correction, such as the removal of an overlapping area, simply pick up the angled interproximal area and rotate it to an upright position. If a large area of the tooth is involved, move part of the tooth using the frame mode.

Cosmetic contouring tips

- When acquiring the image, have your patient place his or her tongue toward the back of the mouth and pose with the arches slightly apart. The darker background will allow you to see a silhouette of the teeth in greater contrast.
- Pay close attention to highlights that occur naturally on the part of the tooth that is closest to the light source. Light reflections suggest a third dimension to the two-dimensional image and can be critical in helping patients visualize proposed changes. You can modify the highlights of the existing teeth by changing the patient's head position when capturing the image. You can also add highlights to show changes in labial anatomy.
- Ideally, the incisal edges of the maxillary teeth follow the contour of the lower lip when the patient smiles (Fig 9-2).

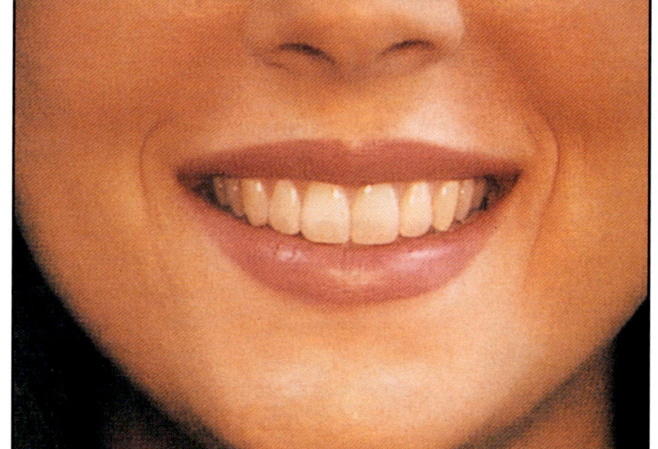

Fig 9-2 When simulating changes to the maxillary anterior teeth, the incisal edges should follow the contour of the lower lip when the patient smiles.

Bleaching

Bleaching, like cosmetic contouring, is a relatively simple treatment that achieves dramatic esthetic improvement in a minimal amount of time. It is also one of the easiest procedures to perform with computer imaging. Bleaching can be accomplished with any view, but shows to best advantage with the patient in full-face smile (Fig 9-3a). Many people think that all they want or need is whiter teeth and are amazed to see that bleaching can actually emphasize existing irregularities. Inform your patient that the colors viewed on the monitor will be a "relative" color and not typically an accurate rendition of the actual tooth color results. If you simulate bleaching first, it will often lead to a discussion of other esthetic changes.

Observe the patient while he or she is smiling and speaking to determine which teeth normally show. Evaluate the smile line. Does the patient show all maxillary teeth or just the span from second bicuspid to second bicuspid? It is not usually necessary to bleach every tooth in each arch; often you may need to bleach only the maxillary teeth, since most patients rarely show the mandibular teeth, with the exception of the incisal edges, when speaking. The easiest way to involve the patient in this decision is to make a short videotape of the patient speaking. Review the tape together and decide which teeth require bleaching. **It is best to bleach one arch at a time so you have the natural unbleached arch of teeth to compare to the bleached teeth.** This will also make it easier to determine how well the bleaching treatment is progressing.

Tooth bleaching may be combined with restorative procedures. For example, before fabricating new anterior crowns or porcelain laminates for your patient, it may be advantageous to first bleach the posterior teeth. You may want to choose a lighter shade for the new prosthetics. Mandibular teeth may be lightened before a restorative shade for the maxillary teeth is selected.

Bleaching tips

- Be sure to diminish the color intensity as teeth regress posteriorly. Remember, posterior teeth usually have shadows and are darker in color. If all the teeth are computer bleached to the same intensity, the imaged smile will appear flat and fake.
- Avoid making the teeth appear too white. Bleach the computer-imaged teeth slightly less than you think you can achieve with the patient's actual teeth to avoid possible disappointment with the clinical results.
- A light-blue or violet wash will reduce the value of very yellow teeth. Pink has the same effect on green, and gray neutralizes yellow.
- If your patient wants only bleaching, yet you feel he or she requires other or additional procedures to achieve the desired effect (eg, cosmetic contouring or laminates), first bleach the teeth as they appear. Your patient may then see the irregularities more vividly, since whiter teeth provide more contrast to the face and will show discrepancies more dramatically. Then consider creating a third image combining all of your suggested changes. Use of this "silent motivator" works well in these situations (see Chapter 10).

While computer systems may differ in their methods for demonstrating bleaching, general guidelines apply:

1. The teeth may be lightened by dragging a brush tip over them in a lighten mode, which blends and lightens simultaneously (Fig 9-3b).
2. Color washes of varying intensities may be applied to the teeth (Fig 9-3c). Usually white is the color of choice, but often a little violet at the incisal edge and a little yellow or yellow-brown at the cervical aspect will produce a more natural result.
3. The polygon tool may be used to illustrate bleaching a group of teeth. The stylus is used to draw borders around the teeth to be bleached, the degree of lightening desired is chosen, and the entire area inside the polygon will be lightened (Fig 9-3d). The result with this polygon technique is that the teeth may look as if the arch has been widened orthodontically. If that is not part of the treatment plan, and it usually will not be, you may inadvertently mislead your patient. This unwanted effect can be minimized by a technique that, in effect, lightens the anterior teeth one shade lighter than the posterior teeth. This reflects the fact that the relative color change of natural teeth after bleaching is usually less as the teeth progress into the buccal corridor.
4. Some systems allow an instant bleach with the touch of a button. The computer can recognize the white of the teeth, as well as the red of the tissue and lips, and will lighten only the teeth.

If your treatment plan includes cosmetic contouring or other reconstructive procedures, image those changes before the bleaching. A restorative simulation will enable you to experiment with varying degrees of bleaching so you can determine which option will look best.

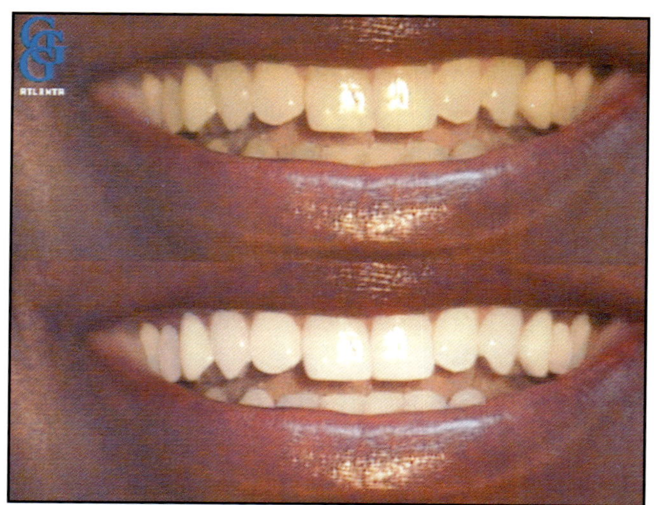

Fig 9-3a Bleaching is another way to achieve dramatic esthetic improvement in a minimal amount of time. The bleaching image can be accomplished using any view, but shows to best advantage in a full face smile.

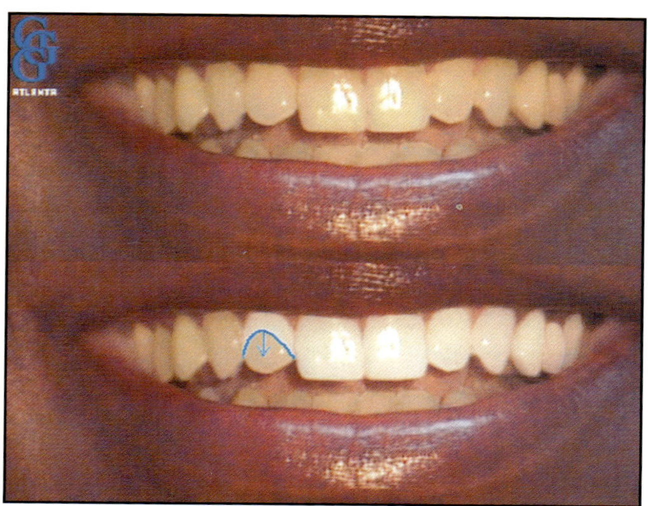

Fig 9-3b The teeth may be lightened by dragging a brush tip over them in a lighten mode, blending and lightening simultaneously.

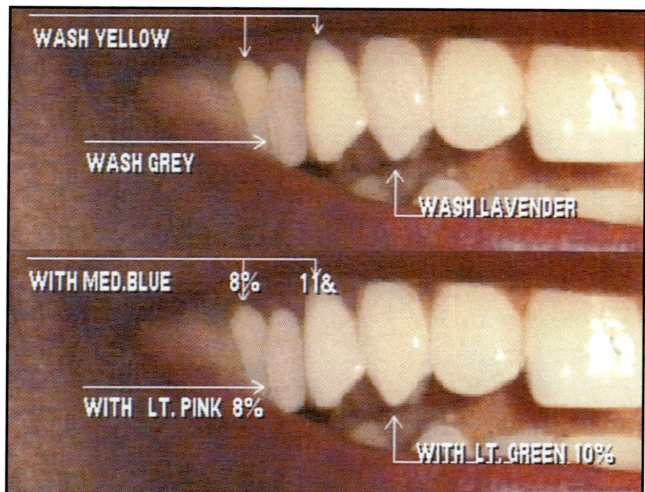

Fig 9-3c The teeth may be lightened by applying color washes or tints of different hues and intensities.

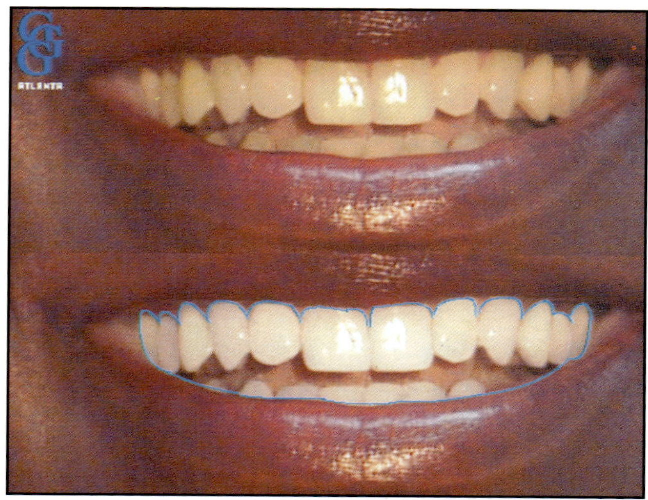

Fig 9-3d The teeth may be "bleached" by outlining the region to be lightened with a polygon tool if available.

Restorative Changes

Restorative procedures such as bonding, laminating, or crowning, which correct fractures, discolorations, spaces, or crowding, will produce esthetic results similar to bleaching or contouring when imaged on the computer. The computer techniques used to simulate these results are also similar.

Lip Line Determination

Many times a patient's lip line will dictate your restorative treatment planning (Fig 9-4a–c). The lip line is important in designing margins for fixed prosthetics and even more so when proposing removable prosthodontics. A high lip line can pose an esthetic challenge for full or partial dentures, and it is a good idea to forewarn your patient if there will be visible clasps. Consider raising gingival margins through various periodontal cosmetic surgical procedures if you can significantly improve your patient's final esthetic results. Previewing this with a computer-imaged try-in is less costly than redesigning a framework and can save valuable laboratory time.

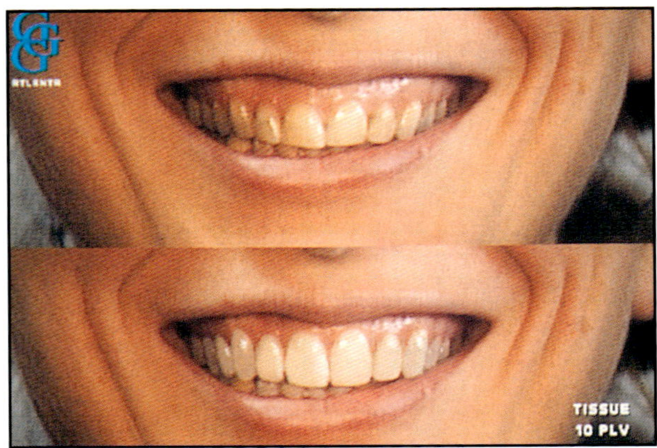

Fig 9-4a High lip line.

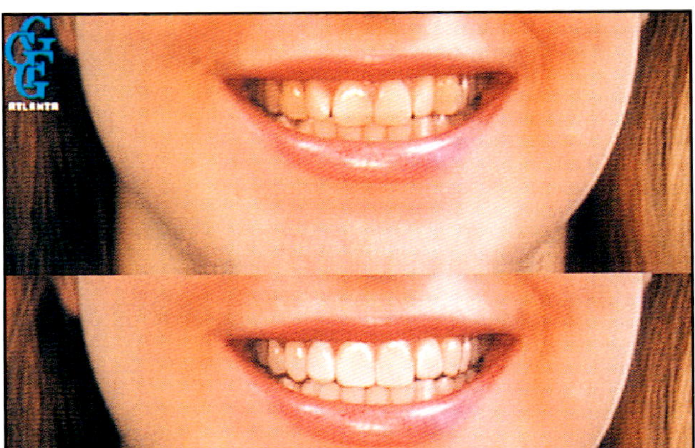

Fig 9-4b Medium lip line.

Fig 9-4a–c A patient's lip line often dictates treatment planning. The lip line is important in designing margins for fixed prostheses and even more so for removable prosthodontics. It is often beneficial to preview and consider raising the gingival margins and/or an orthognathic correction before restorative or esthetic treatments.

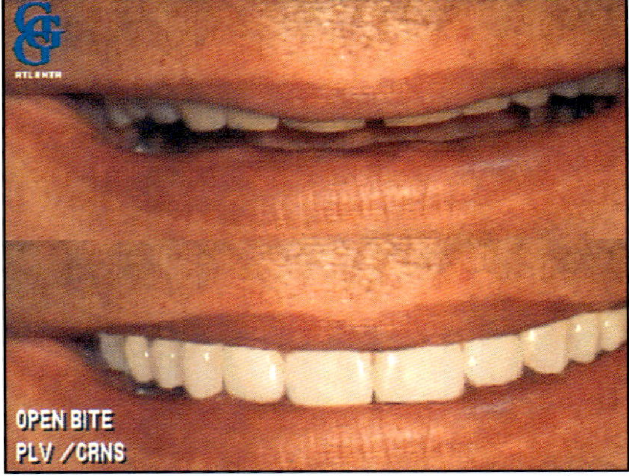

Fig 9-4c Low lip line.

Replacing Amalgam Restorations

Patients may request replacement of their amalgam restorations with tooth-colored materials. As a result, the tooth shade as seen from the buccal view will appear somewhat lighter when the amalgam is replaced. (If the buccal color does not sufficiently improve, you may recommend a porcelain laminate or full-coverage restoration).

1. If the restoration is not large, color can be drawn ("dragged") over the cusps toward the central fossa; take care not to obscure the anatomy.
2. Pay attention to the facial sides of amalgam-stained teeth. If it is not possible to blend out the discoloration, you may need to move tooth color from another part of the tooth or from an adjacent tooth (Fig 9-5).
3. If the restoration is extensive, use a tooth from another part of the arch, select one from the tooth bank, or show your patient an actual before-and-after case from a computerized album.

Placing/Replacing Composites

1. When imaging composite restorations, eliminate any telltale discolored margins or surfaces.
2. Usually, you can achieve a more natural result by moving an appropriately sized portion from another tooth to the unesthetic area by using a cut-and-paste move (Fig 9-6).
3. Color can be "pulled" over the area to be restored, although the result may appear smeared or flat. (Horizontal strokes work better than vertical ones) (Fig 9-7).

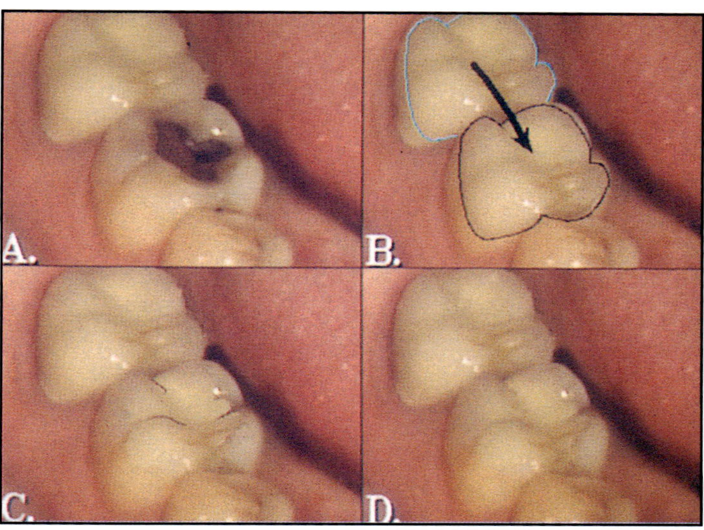

Fig 9-5 Amalgam replacement can be effectively simulated by using a tooth from elsewhere in the patient's arch or by selecting an appropriate tooth from the library.

Labial Veneering

Technically, it will be difficult to tell whether a computer image represents a direct bonded veneer or a porcelain laminate. However, full facial bonding usually creates a thicker, rounder tooth (especially if the tooth is not prepared [Fig 9-8a]), with highlights in different areas (the center). Use existing teeth for the image when possible, or select teeth from the tooth bank, to obtain the desired shade and shape (Fig 9-9).

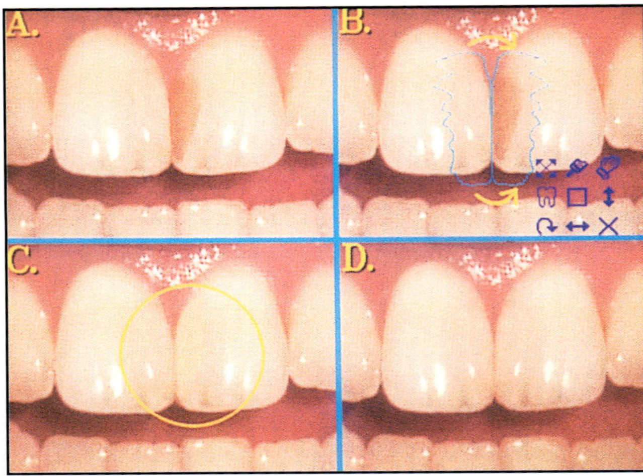

Fig 9-6 A, This stained composite requires replacement. B, A section of a similar tooth is outlined, moved, flipped, and pasted over the stained composite. C and D, The added area is now blended, and a proper light reflection is placed to show depth.

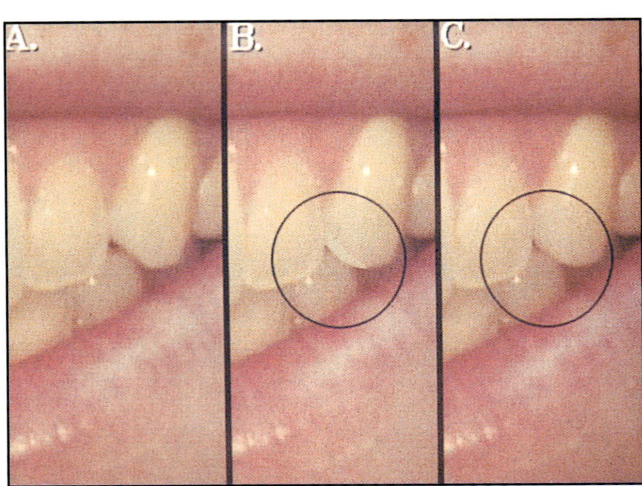

Fig 9-7 A, The mesial embrasure of this cuspid requires closing. B, A color is chosen from the area and is "dragged" over the area to be closed. C, The area is now blended.

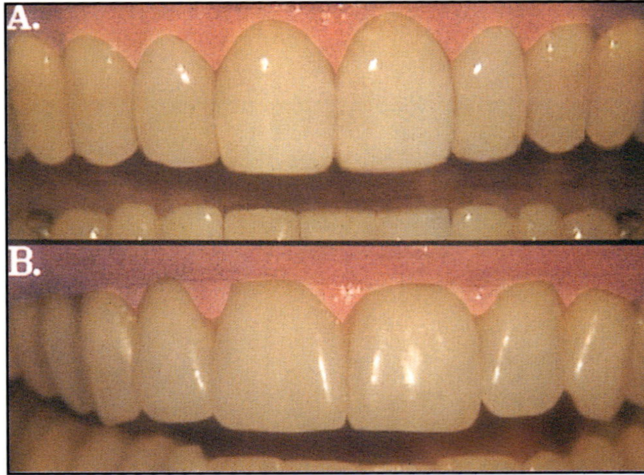

Fig 9-8 A, Full facial bonding often appears bulky and with rounded facial contours. B, Laminate veneers usually provide a more natural appearance.

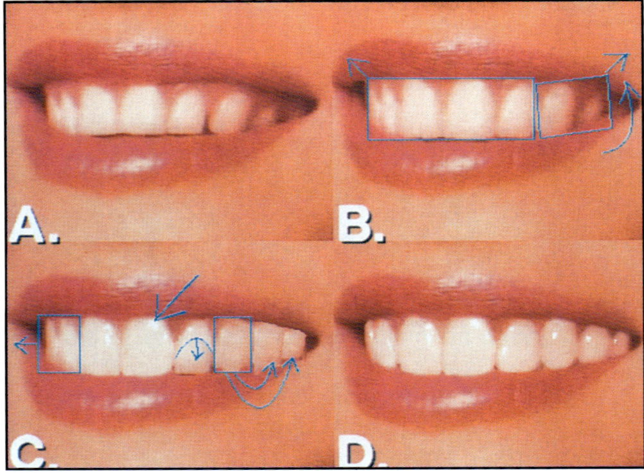

Fig 9-9 This laminate veneer simulation was created by using framed moves to lengthen and widen the patient's natural teeth and raise the tissue. The buccal vestibules are filled and the teeth bleached.

Restorative tips

- Highlights occur where the tooth is closest to the light. Bonding highlights tend to be toward the center of the tooth (see Fig 9-8a).
- Crown and porcelain laminate veneer highlights often occur on edges and line angles, giving the tooth a flatter look (see Fig 9-8b).
- Subtle highlights from a natural tooth can be repositioned to your imaged tooth.

Line Angles. Line angles can be an important factor for achieving tooth harmony in the arch. Tooth line angles occur where surface planes change direction. The mesial line angle occurs where the facial surface meets the mesial surface. Distal line angles are created by the meeting of the facial and distal surfaces of the tooth.

Tooth highlights often occur along line angles because that aspect of the tooth is nearest to the light source. An arch in harmony will present a regular pattern of mesial line angles (Fig 9-10a). Teeth out of alignment will exhibit irregular angles and an irregular pattern of light reflection (Fig 9-10b).

The angles will increase progressively around the arch from anterior teeth to posterior teeth, which tend to have a more triangular silhouette. The line angles on a central incisor are nearly parallel to its long axis. An understanding of line angles can provide helpful guidance for imaging any changes affecting alignment of the teeth. Adding appropriately placed highlights to the image on the line angles can help your patient visualize the intended result more accurately.

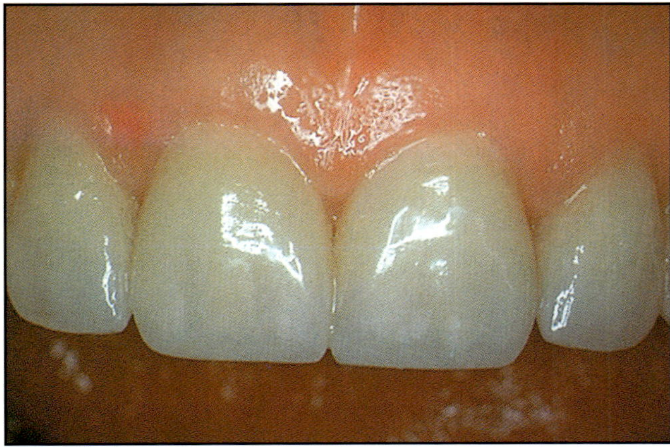

Fig 9-10a Line angles can be an important factor for determining tooth harmony in the dental arch. An anterior segment that is in harmony will present a regular pattern of mesial line angles and light reflection.

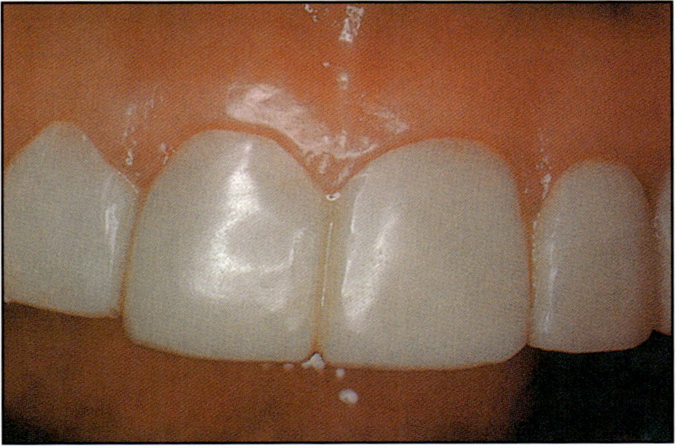

Fig 9-10b Teeth out of alignment exhibit irregular line angles and light reflection patterns. An understanding of line angles can provide helpful guidance for imaging changes affecting the alignment of the teeth.

Crown Restorations

Since the full-crown restoration provides the greatest latitude in esthetic correction, tooth position will be the chief limiting factor. Try to coordinate your imaging simulations with the diagnostic study casts to see how much correction you can accomplish. Whether crowns are fabricated of metal and porcelain, or of just porcelain or resin, they will image with a similar result (Fig 9-11a and b).

The extent of the intended change will determine the best tool to image the alterations. Usually, a cut-and-paste move is best. In the case of multiple crowns, however, it may be easier to use teeth from a tooth bank.

Crown restoration tips

- If the final crowns will have metal labial and or lingual collars, show a larger metal collar than needed. This will help to ensure that your patient understands the intended result.
- Use your simulations to communicate with your lab technician. The images are invaluable in enhancing communication and aiding the technician in all aspects of provisional and final restoration fabrication.

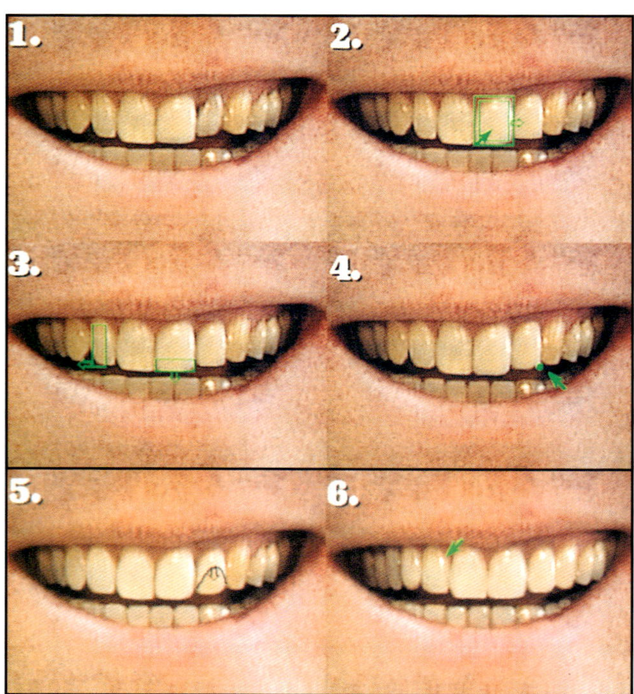

Fig 9-11a 1, This patient requires a new bridge. 2, The central incisor is reduced, then cut and pasted into the pontic position. 3, The central is lengthened; the lateral is widened. 4, The incisal edges are contoured. 5, The teeth are bleached. 6, Correct highlights are added to the teeth.

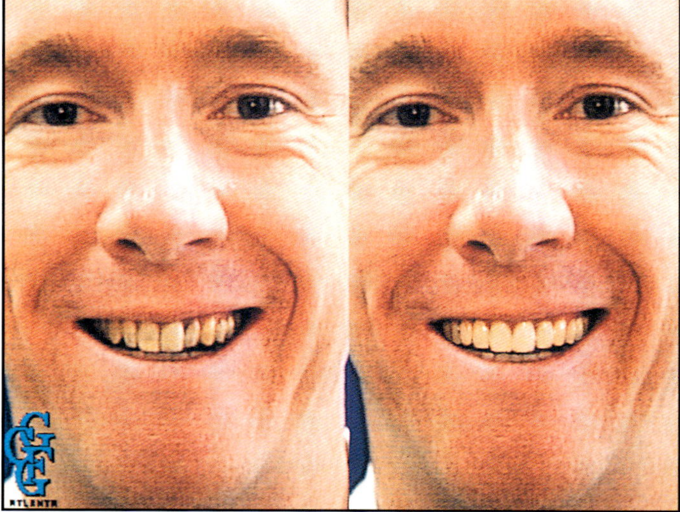

Fig 9-11b The before-and-after full-face images.

Fixed Prostheses

Computer imaging is advantageous for space measurement to ensure that the replacement tooth or teeth will look proportionate (Fig 9-12). Replacing a tooth through imaging can be accomplished by "flipping" a tooth from the other side of the arch (Fig 9-13). If that is not possible, select a tooth with the appropriate color and silhouette form from the tooth bank. In either case, you may need to reposition or contour the teeth to make them fit into the space properly. If the area around a pontic does not look natural, consider showing a ridge augmentation (Fig 9-14).

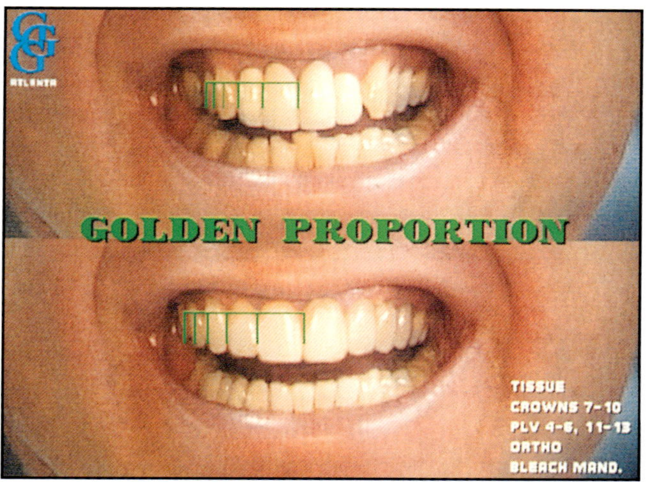

Fig 9-12 When new prosthetics are needed, computer imaging is helpful in measuring and demonstrating to patients the result of better tooth sizing.

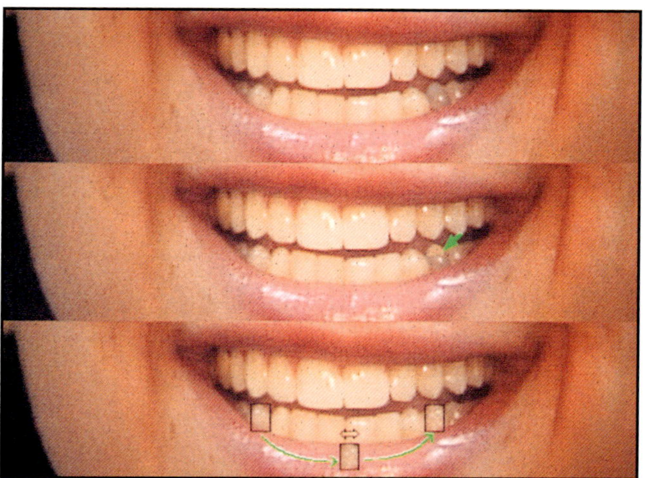

Fig 9-13 The dark lower bicuspid needs replacement. The bicuspid from the opposite side of the arch is cut, pasted, and flipped.

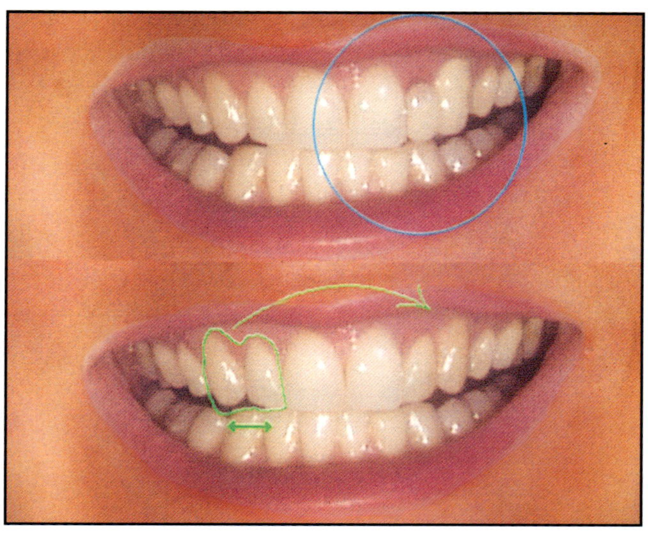

Fig 9-14 When pontic areas appear false, the opposite arch may be cut, pasted, and flipped to provide an esthetic alternative.

Try-in

Normally, when a patient arrives for the try-in of porcelain crowns or laminates, the restorations are placed temporarily into the mouth and evaluated for fit, function, and color. Necessary adjustments are made by adding or subtracting material. However, it may be more effective to image the patient at try-in. Use the computer to check the restorations and to evaluate for the various esthetic criteria such as tooth length, width, form, etc. This saves much time and effort.

Imaging lets you see where to add or subtract from the restorations. You can also examine the color and decide whether to lighten or darken and whether cervical color or incisal translucency is needed. You can evaluate the buccal corridor and the smile line. **The computer gives you a second chance to make alterations.**

Most importantly, imaging allows your patient to preview their new restorations before they are cemented. Remaking restorations due to esthetic misinterpretations can be costly.

Esthetic checklist

1. Smile line—high, medium, low
2. Tooth length
3. Tissue—contour, texture, color
4. Buccal corridor—wide (arch appears narrow); thin (arch appears broad)
5. Size—golden proportion
6. Shape of teeth—triangular, rounded, square
7. Facial contour—rounded or flat
8. Facial and incisal embrasures—opened to show tooth individuality
9. Line angles, light reflections, highlights
10. Rounded corners
11. Surface texture—lines of imbrication, lobes
12. Tooth color
13. Cervical color
14. Incisal halo
15. Smooth color transition
16. Check lines or cracks

Prosthetic Planning

For patients who require full-mouth restoration or denture fabrication, it may be best to choose teeth from the tooth bank (see Chapter 8). Carefully align the smiles, one over the other, and check the alignment with vertical lines (see page 91). Pictures of the patient's natural teeth can guide your selection of tooth size and shape and reveal how much of the teeth show when the patient smiles.

Periodontal Esthetics

One of the more recent changes in esthetic dentistry has been the increasing use of periodontal surgery to enhance dentofacial harmony. The generalist and public alike are recognizing the remarkable improvements that can be achieved when the teeth, the gingival soft-tissue profiles, and the lip form are in harmony. Imaging can be an invaluable aid to help patients visualize the esthetic potential for plastic surgical procedures such as "gum raising." Only when they see computer-altered images with the incorporated changes can patients fully appreciate their value.

Similarly, imaging can help you and your patient decide on the best approach to a case by enabling you to try alternative treatments on the screen. In a high lip-line case, for instance, you can see whether periodontal surgery will suffice or if orthognathic surgery will be necessary (Fig 9-15).

Images for the esthetic diagnosis of smile harmony should include frontal views of the full face in repose and smiling, especially for patients who show a lot of tissue in a full smile and little or no teeth in repose. Close-up views of both the normal smile and the forced wide smile or grimace are also required. Close-up views of the arches (with the lips retracted) are essential for surgical cosmetic treatment planning.

Once you and the patient have agreed on a course of treatment, print hard copies of the computer-imaged changes for the patient and/or chart (Fig 9-16). These prints will eliminate guesswork and can serve as a useful guide during the surgical procedure (Fig 9-17).

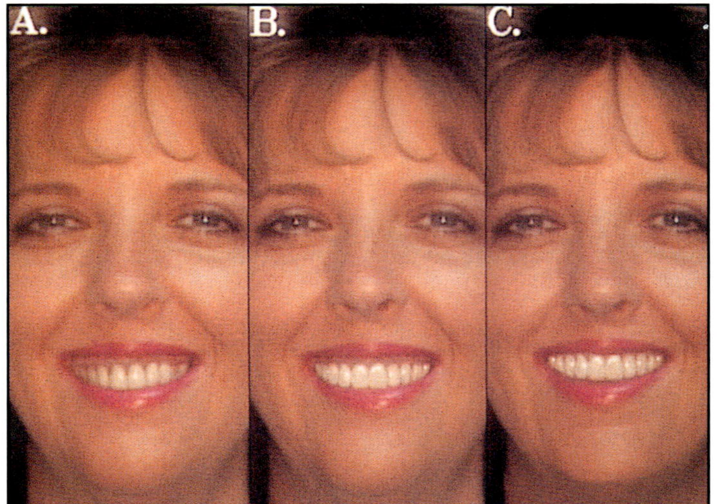

Fig 9-15 A, This young woman seeks esthetic improvement. B, Imaging shows how her smile will appear after esthetic tissue surgery and new crowns. C, A different, possibly more esthetic, alternative entails the use of orthognathic surgery.

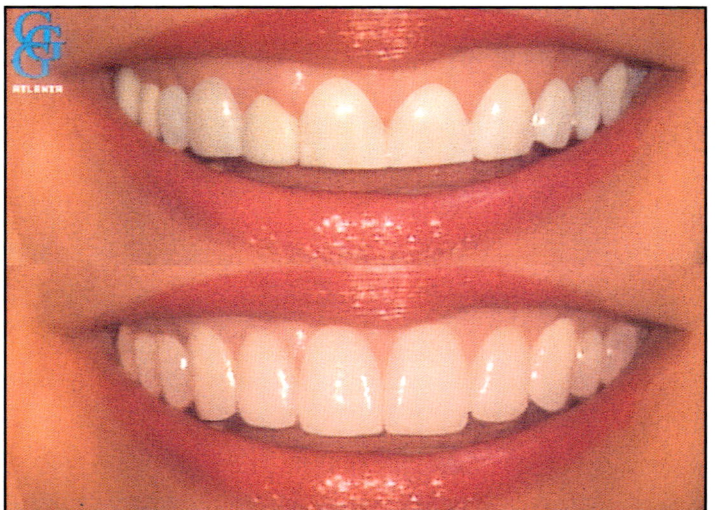

Fig 9-16 This before-and-after image is useful for both the patient and the referral source.

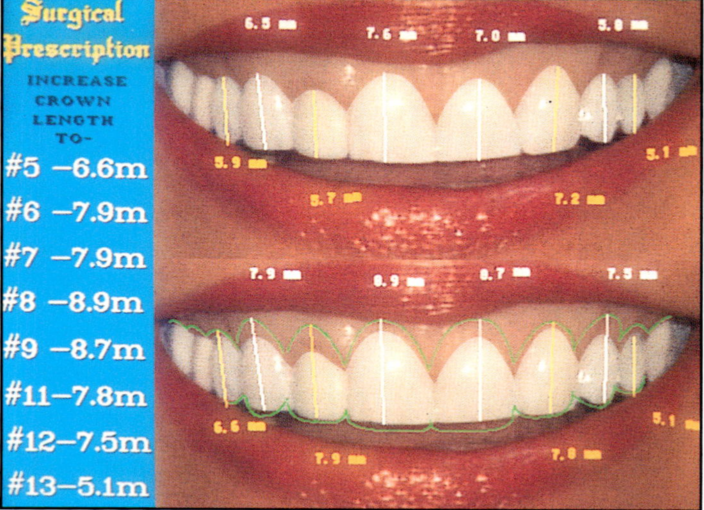

Fig 9-17 A surgical prescription image is essential to send to your referral source.

Gingival Recontouring

There are several ways to simulate the esthetic effects of routine periodontal flap procedures to improve a "gummy" smile. However, the feasibility of imaged changes must be determined based on factors including root length, occlusal relationships, osseous trabecular pattern, incisal guidance, and crown emergence profile with close root proximity.

1. Frame part of the tooth from the mid-point to the cervical margin and move it apically to the desired height (Fig 9-18a and b).
2. Contour and blend in the cervical edge as required (Fig 9-18c).
3. Contour the incisal edges to parallel the arch of the lower lip (Fig 9-18d) and alter the color as necessary.

The dimensions of any aspect of a tooth can be superimposed over the on-screen image. The computer can then extrapolate all other dimensions. Imaging systems that incorporate a measurement package will set a scale to one tooth so that all other measurements will be in relative proportion.

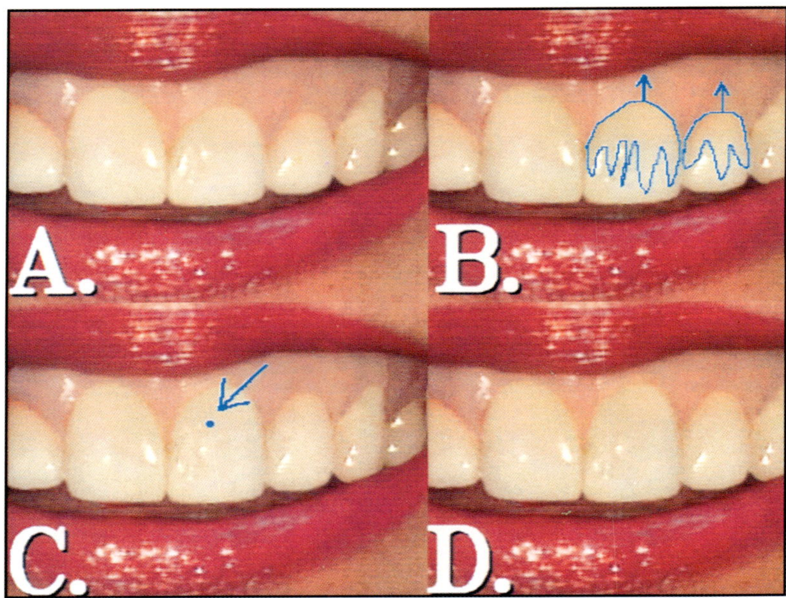

Fig 9-18 A, A high lip line and an abundance of gingival display is a common esthetic problem. B, To simulate a reduction of gingival display, frame the teeth from the midpoint to just above the gingival margin and move the polygon apically to the desired height. C, Contour and blend the cervical aspects of the teeth. D, The final result.

Gingival recontouring tips

- The central incisors and cuspids will usually be approximately the same length from the incisal edge. The lateral incisors will be slightly shorter, at both the cervical and the incisal aspects (Fig 9-19a).
- Remember, that *clinically* the tooth and root will become thinner as more tissue and bone are removed. Consequently, the final result may have blunted papillae and small dark triangles of missing interproximal tissue ("black triangle disease"). These areas can be filled with porcelain. Pink or tissue-colored porcelains often will appear more natural looking, especially with medium and low lip-line patients. Tooth-colored porcelain may result in wider, squarer teeth, especially at the cervical aspects. Another option is a tissue stent (Fig 9-19b)
- Evaluate the bicuspid area, as short bicuspids often detract from the smile. Usually this is evident from a frontal view, but oblique views help the patient see the area more clearly. Raise the bicuspids to the same level as the anterior teeth by capturing part of the tooth from midpoint to cervical and moving it apically (Fig 9-20).
- A ridge augmentation can be imaged by moving tissue from a normal area close by into the recessed area or by flipping the contralateral tooth and tissue (Fig 9-21).
- Remember, the lips may have to be repositioned using the copy or duplicate function if a section of the lip is obliterated during the process.
- Be aware that the line angles of the teeth may need to be repositioned to achieve a natural-looking result.

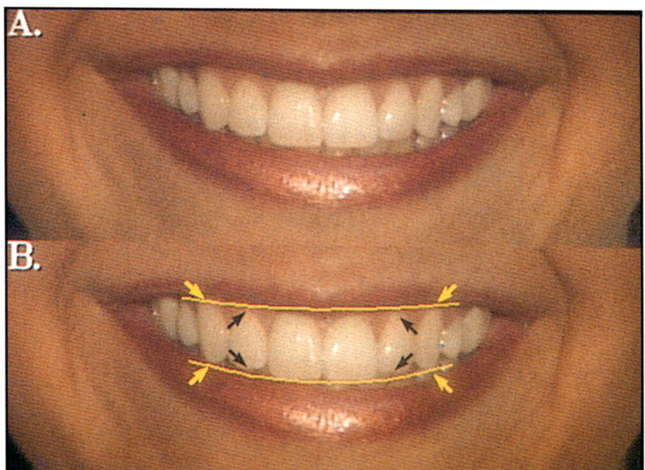

Fig 9-19a When working with the tissue, the central incisors and cuspids should be the same length and the lateral incisors shorter.

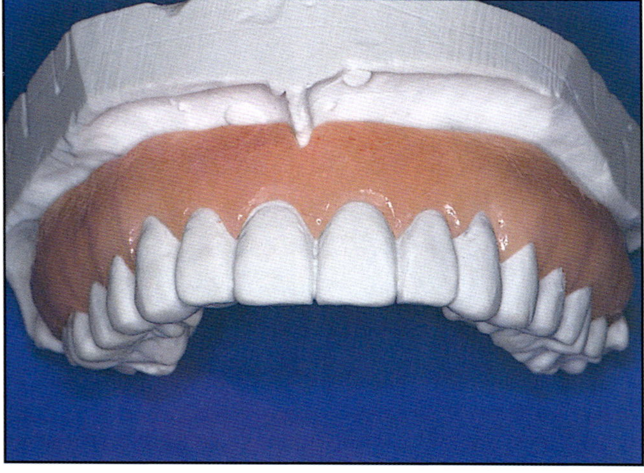

Fig 9-19b A removable acrylic tissue stent is a viable option for certain patients who have lost interdental tissue, resulting in unattractive open spaces.

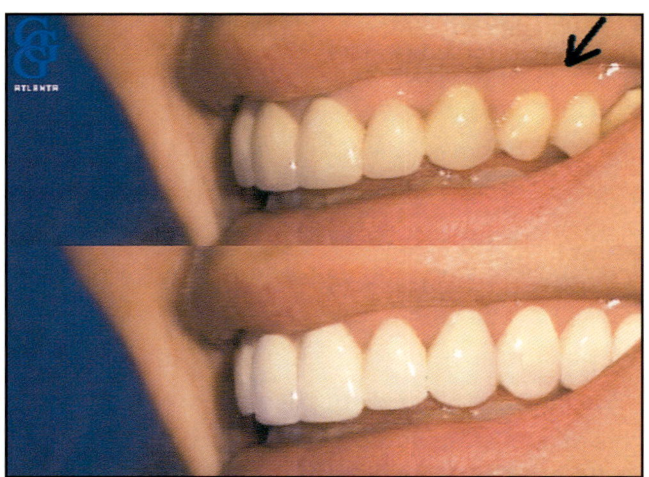

Fig 9-20 Excessive tissue and short clinical crowns in the bicuspid regions must also be addressed.

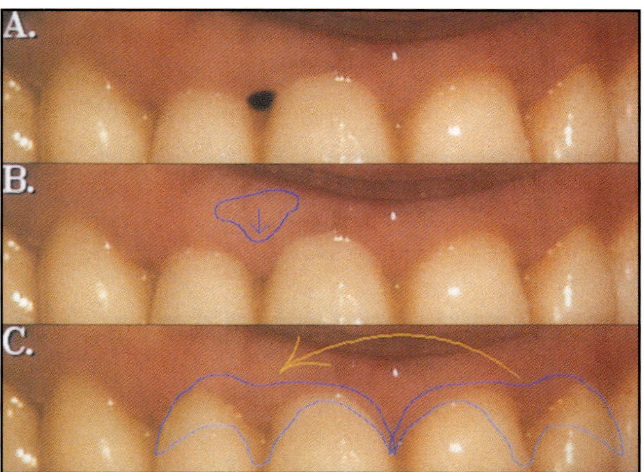

Fig 9-21 A, Unesthetic "black triangle disease" should be corrected. B, A portion of healthy tissue may be "dragged" into the area. C, Alternatively, tissue from the contralateral side may be used.

Orthodontics

The illustrative capabilities of computer imaging can be particularly useful to patients who are embarking on a course of orthodontic treatment. Patients can visualize not only the treatment goals, but also how various types of orthodontic appliances will appear on their teeth during treatment (Fig 9-22 and 9-23). Computer imaging makes the whole process less of a mystery, especially when it is accomplished in organized stages.

Progressive Imaging

This technique can provide your patients with accurate and finely tuned results. Progressive imaging involves three tiers.

Baseline/Projected Images. These initial pictures show the patient's current malocclusion and provide an image of what you seek to achieve with orthodontic therapy.

Interim/Pre-Bracket Removal Imaging. Imaging the patient before the brackets are removed provides an opportunity to evaluate the intended orthodontic outcome (Fig 9-24a). The posterior dentition of the patient shown in Fig 9-24b, for example, is still lingually inclined, which would leave her with an unattractive smile. Make a print-out and send it to the orthodontist so that the proper changes can be made. After viewing these images, the attending orthodontist may recommend extending treatment to accomplish an important change in the patient's final appearance.

You can better analyze spacing before restorative treatment by removing brackets on the computer. Measure or use the golden proportion to determine if the teeth are properly positioned and can be restored to proper proportion to avoid surprises once the brackets are removed (Fig 9-24c).

On the other hand, the general dentist who is completing prosthetic treatment may want the teeth in slight linguoversion, for instance, to minimize the amount of tooth reduction necessary to accommodate laminates (Fig 9-24b) for anterior teeth. Typically, the cervical will be correctly positioned and need to be prepared for a laminate. But leaving the anterior teeth properly in linguoversion may require little or no facial reduction, except a slight chamfer around the periphery of the tooth, since this aspect of the tooth will be laminated with at least 1.0 mm to 1.5 mm of porcelain.

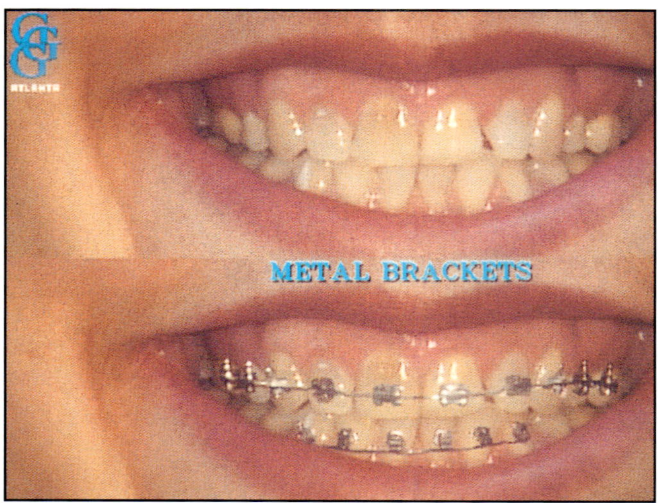

Fig 9-22 A patient imaged with metal brackets.

Fig 9-23 A computer image can be used to show your patient the esthetic difference between metal and porcelain bracketing.

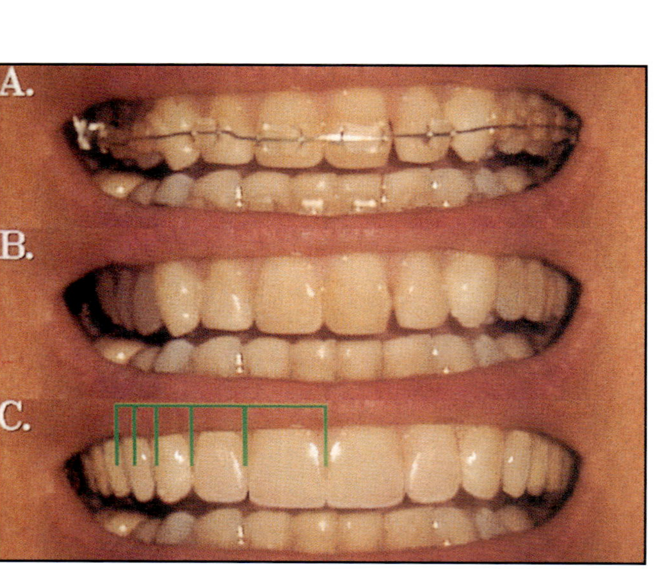

Fig 9-24 A, This patient has been told her brackets are ready for removal. A pre-bracket-removal visit allows verification of the orthodontic result before the brackets are clinically removed. B, The computer image shows the patient's dentition with the brackets removed. Notice the unesthetic outcome of the posterior dentition. C, The golden proportion grid enables analysis to determine if the orthodontic result will allow proper positioning of new restorations.

Final Imaging. Once the brackets are removed, you may decide to alter your initial projected restorative treatment plan. Now is the best time to communicate this with your patient. The three-tiered progressive imaging approach helps your patients understand their treatment alterations. Naturally, this process will involve more time and visits with the imaging technician, and the costs involved should be reflected in your fees.

The Technique. The frontal view can show the proposed treatment and expected results to the patients. A full face with a wide smile is helpful also to illustrate the intended tooth and gingival changes; a close-up smile is indicated for some patients, especially when tooth size discrepancies are present.

1. Slightly crowded teeth can be moved one by one (Fig 9-25) or in groups, rotating them when necessary.
2. In some situations, it may be easier to move teeth from one side of the arch to the other, for example, by flipping over tooth 8 and moving it into the 9 position (Fig 9-26).
3. Overlapping incisal or cervical ends of teeth can be changed by framing the teeth from mid-tooth to the desired apical or incisal edge as needed.
4. Incisal edges can also be reshaped using the tongue color, as in cosmetic contouring.
5. When proposed changes are extensive, it is quicker to choose a set of straight teeth from the tooth bank and insert them into the image.
6. When moving teeth or tissue, you may obscure an area accidentally. Different systems offer different solutions. On some systems, the original image may be restored with the correct mouse button; on others, the best way to restore part of the original image is with the copy mode, which allows you to retrieve unaltered portions from the original image. Still other systems use different options.

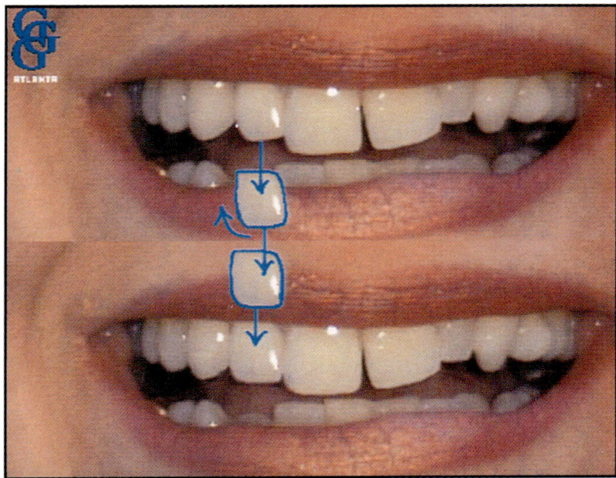

Fig 9-25 Outline the malaligned tooth and rotate it until it appears correctly positioned in the arch.

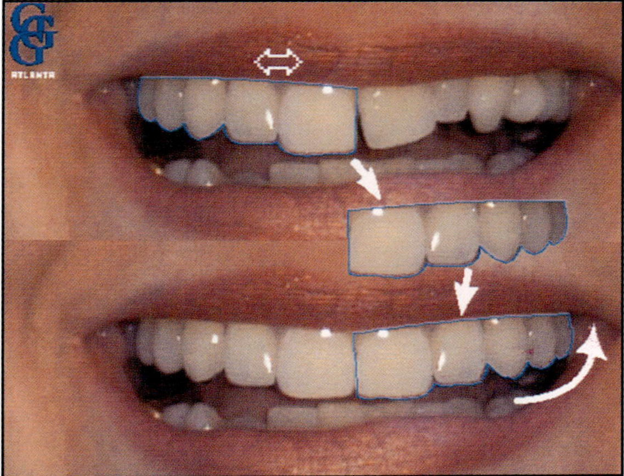

Fig 9-26 Often, outlining one side of the arch and flipping it will provide a nice approximation of an orthodontic result.

Maxillofacial Surgery

Because patients may approach surgery with understandable reluctance, computer imaging can have a most dramatic effect in convincing them of the need for surgery. Most patients are amazed when they see the impact surgery can have on their appearance and are eager to do whatever is necessary to achieve the results. Imaging allows the patient and doctor to decide what the extent of the correction should be and to plan treatment accordingly. Questions about additional cosmetic changes, such as whether to surgically alter the chin or nose, may arise during consultation; these, too, can be explored through imaging.

The profile view is generally best to demonstrate projected surgical changes (Fig 9-27), although a full-face and/or oblique view may be needed for frontal deformities (Fig 9-28). Plotted movements can be shown on a cephalometric image, image profile, or both (Fig 9-29). Specialized software is available to enable you to portray tissue relocation on the video profile coordinated with the predictive tracing on the electronic cephalograph.

Like the cephalometric radiograph, the computer image should be captured without the patient smiling. Be sure to include a ruler or other measuring device in the image; this will enable you to properly calibrate the computer's measuring scale.

Maxillofacial surgery tips

- Moving the mandible forward will tighten tissue under the chin, unless the surgeon compensates by surgically reducing the chin. Moving the mandible back usually results in a more defined lower lip and a deeper indentation under the lip.
- If orthodontic, orthognathic, and plastic surgery treatments are to be integrated, obtain the patient's frontal and profile images with and without a smile, so that tooth relationships can be shown.
- Some surgeons like additional lateral views as well as a view of the mouth at rest, which shows the lip-tooth relationships. Consult with the involved surgeons to ensure that you provide the images they need.

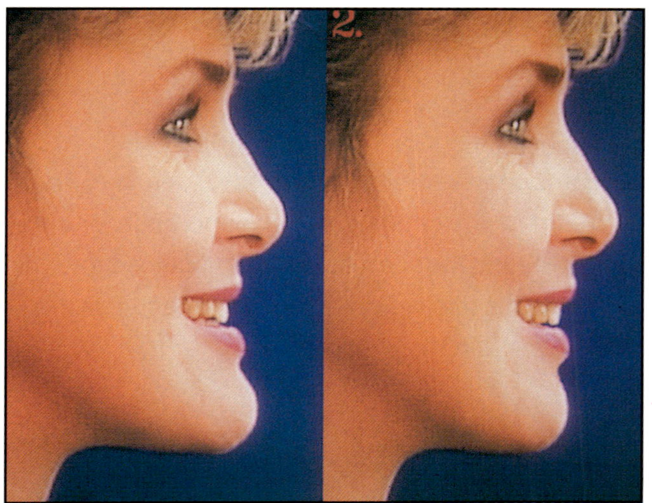

Fig 9-27 A profile view is often best suited to show potential results of surgery.

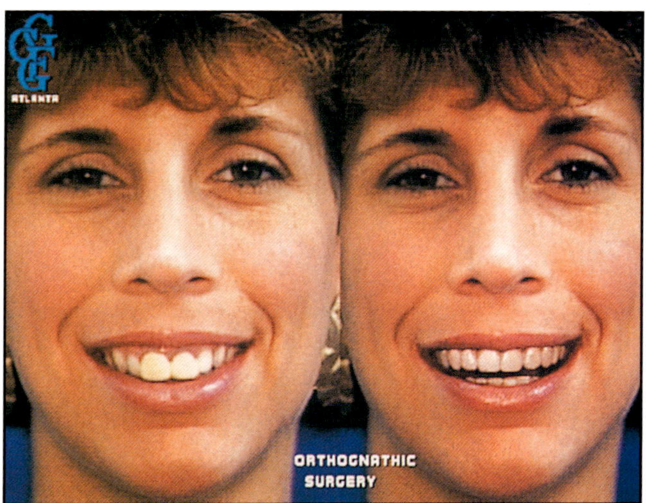

Fig 9-28 The full face view is best to depict frontal changes.

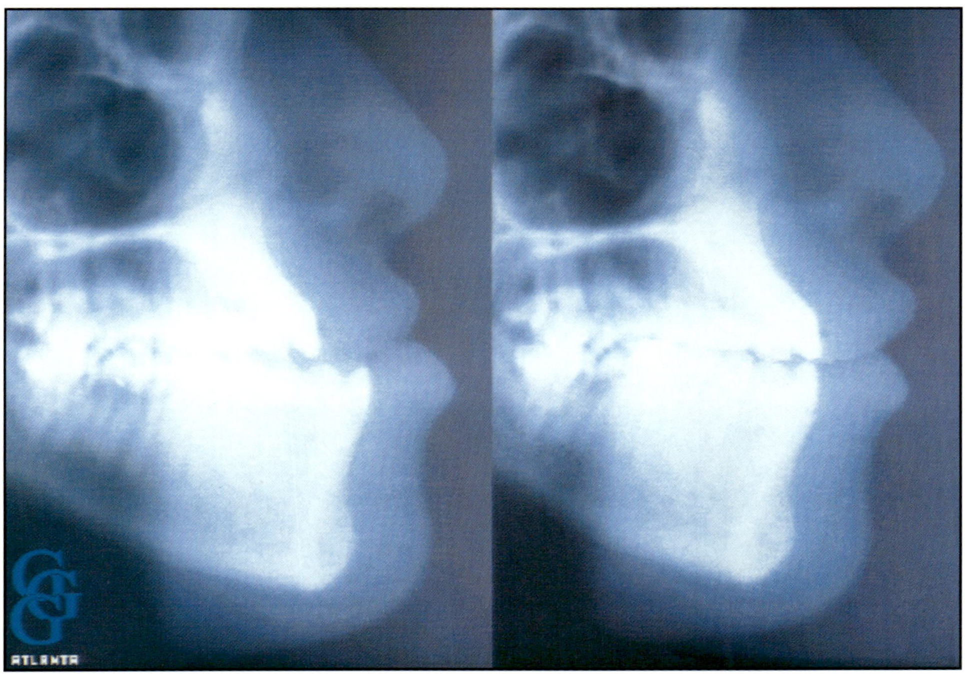

Fig 9-29 Note the planned movement on this cephalometric image.

Implants

Many patients are reluctant to consider implants for their treatment plan because they are unaware of implant improvements or how they are used. The computer can image an MRI, a CT scan, or a cephalometric, panoramic, or intraoral radiograph (Figs 9-30 to 9-32); the implant can be sized and placed into the radiograph with the use of a window. This allows your patient to see the size of the implant and where it would be placed in the mouth.

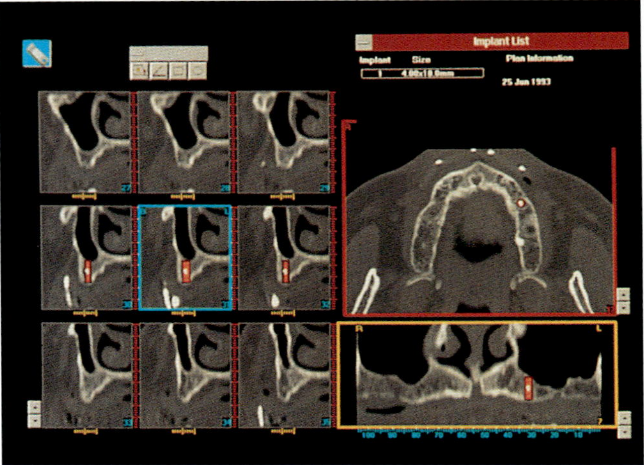

Fig 9-30 This computed tomographic scan image is used to evaluate proper bone contour and consistency for placement of implants. (SIM/Plant, Columbia Scientific)

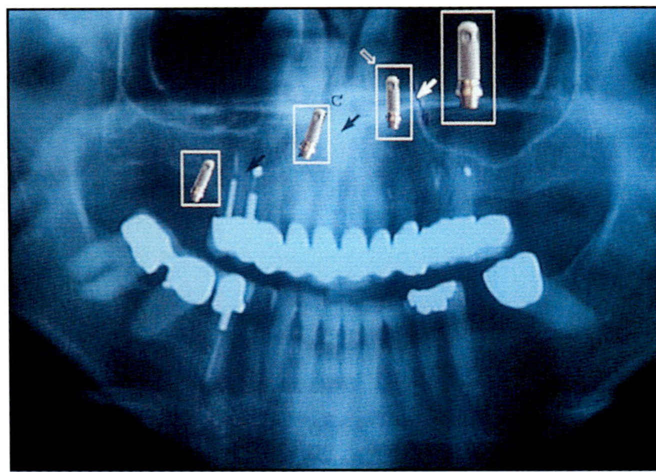

Fig 9-31 Patients may find it easier to understand implant placement when viewing a Panorex image.

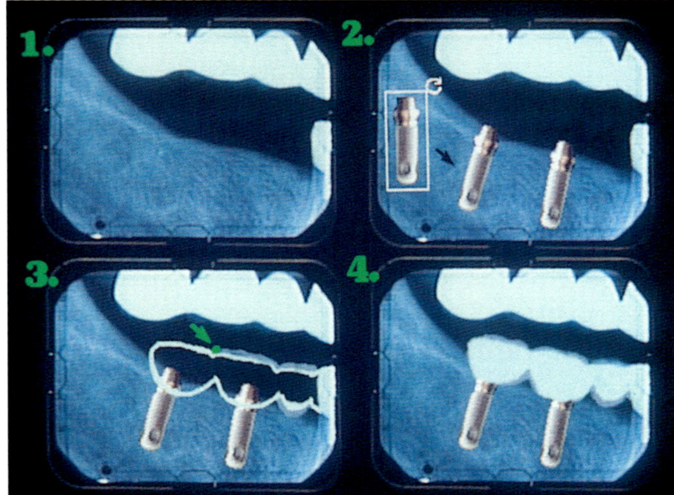

Fig 9-32 Intraoral radiographs are also useful in showing a patient's implant placement.

A similar procedure can be done using an image of the patient's mouth. The top of the implant and the transmucosal insert can be brought into the image with a window to show the patient how the implant will be placed. Next, a replacement tooth can be imaged over the implant to give your patient a complete picture of the procedure (Fig 9-33).

These procedures can also improve communication among the surgeon, the restorative dentist, and the technician. The image can show the projected final appearance of the prosthesis, and everyone on the treatment team can evaluate the restorative outcome of any compromises in fixture placement. It is also helpful, once the implants are placed and the prosthetic stage is planned, to image a postoperative radiograph of the implants and an intraoral view of the transmucosal inserts. Planning through imaging can save valuable technician hours.

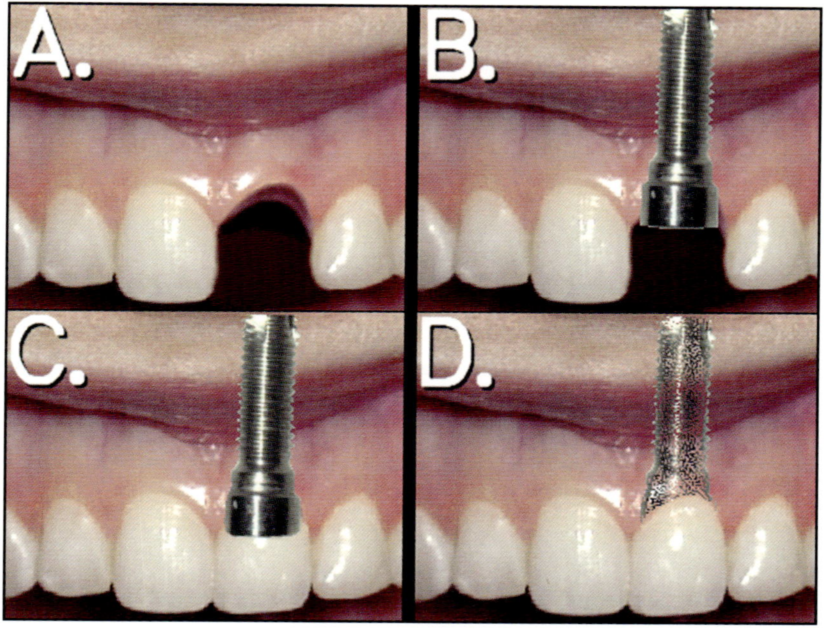

Fig 9-33 This image depicts implant placement and restoration for patients.

Reference

1. Goldstein RE. Esthetics in Dentistry. Toronto: BC Decker, 1998.

Preventing *Esthetic* Failures

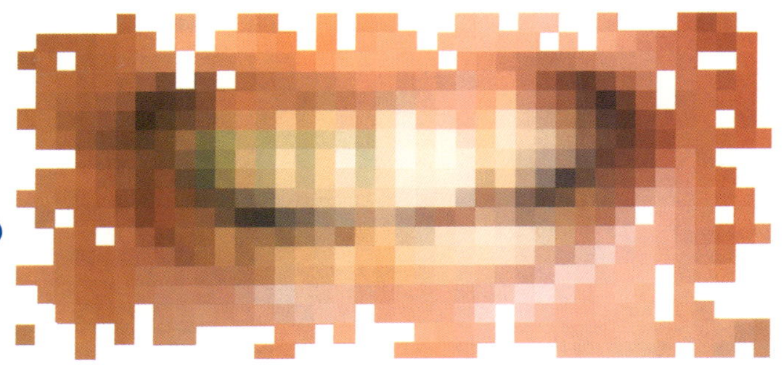

10

Esthetic failure, as well as the failure to meet patient expectations, is costly to everyone in terms of time, money, and emotional well-being. No one disputes that good communication is an important key to preventing failure that may be devastating, even irreversible.

Computer imaging can be an integral part of a diagnostic and treatment protocol that will minimize the chance of miscommunication. The use of imaging at the various stages of diagnosis, treatment planning, case presentation, try-in, and final therapy can improve your expectations of esthetic success and patient satisfaction.

Computer imaging can be an integral part of a diagnostic and treatment protocol that will minimize the chance of miscommunication.

Diagnosis

Computer imaging is highly personalized. The patient can understand your observations and proposed treatment if he or she can see the situation on an image of his or her own face and mouth. Imaging presents a comprehensive range of views, such as a profile smile, that exposes problems the patients probably have never seen or imagined. While seeing these problems may be disconcerting at first, most patients eventually are gratified to learn of, and have the opportunity to correct, any defects. Patient awareness is the first step in therapy, and nothing can help bring a patient to that threshold better and faster than a caring dentist using computer imaging technology.

Computer imaging allows you and the patient to easily consider all pertinent treatment options, including integrated therapies. Patient feedback can help to refine acceptable options to include in the treatment planning phase,

Imaging and diagnosis	
Patient advantages	**Doctor advantages**
See different views	Visualize treatment options
Discover "hidden" problems	Improve patient confidence
See actual image rather than reversed image	Medical-legal documentation

saving time and reducing guesswork. An additional benefit is that you have excellent medical and legal documentation of the patient's original condition and your diagnostic process.

Treatment Planning

Individualized treatment planning is the next phase in preventing esthetic failures. Some of the steps in treatment planning may include:

1. Evaluating the smile line
2. Verifying the need for the golden proportion
3. Providing treatment options
4. Supplying specialty prescriptions to your referral doctors

An initial esthetic treatment plan for your patient may involve the coordination of different subspecialties of dentistry. Restorative dentistry, prosthodontics, periodontics, orthodontics, and orthognathic surgery may be needed in differing degrees to achieve esthetic harmony. For example, Figure 10-1 shows an unesthetic bridge: this man's arch should be widened by orthodontics, the tissue grafted and sculpted by periodontics, and the teeth enlarged by prosthodontics to provide an esthetic smile.

When evaluating a patient's smile, note the length of the teeth. Do they follow the contour of the lower lip? Are the central incisors longer than the laterals; are they even with the cuspids? Does your patient have a high, medium, or low lip line? A high lip line usually necessitates porcelain labial margins, which can decrease the possibility of esthetic success. There are numerous other points to evaluate in your patient's smile; page 104 provides a detailed esthetic checklist.

The golden proportion discussed in the last chapter should be considered when planning for tooth resizing. This is also the ideal time to determine if orthodontic therapy is necessary to correctly reposition the teeth (Fig 10-1, bottom).

The computer allows you to explore and question treatment options easily and quickly: Is a bridge, a partial, or even an implant the more appropriate restoration for missing anterior teeth? Will cosmetic contouring provide the result your patient is seeking? Let the possibility of esthetic failure or disappointment happen on the computer, not in the patient's mouth!

Once the treatment plan is presented and accepted (with the patient's signature), you have accurate pictorial documentation with which to communicate to your staff, the laboratory technician, and, if appropriate, referring doctors (Fig 10-2).

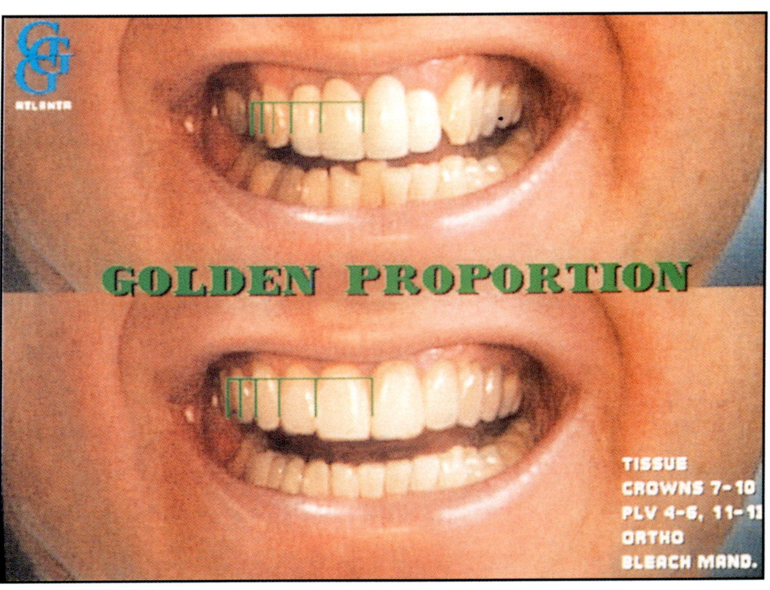

Fig 10-1 *Top, This patient seeks esthetic improvement by replacing the bridge. Bottom, Thorough evaluation and esthetic imaging indicate that bridge replacement and other therapies are necessary to improve the smile.*

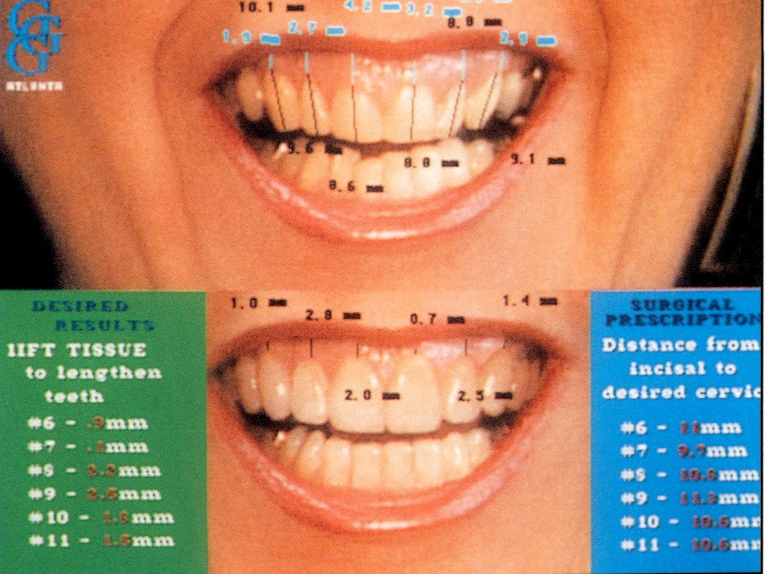

Fig 10-2 *This image shows in detail to the referral dentist the corrections necessary for this smile.*

Imaging and treatment planning

Patient advantages	Doctor advantages
Less expensive	Fewer diagnostic tools needed
Less in-office time	Rapid evaluation of options
Easier to understand	Specialty prescriptions produced
Confident decision making	

Treatment Plan Presentation

Many patients requesting esthetic enhancement are unable to accurately describe the results they expect. However, patients often have a treatment plan in mind when they consult with you. That plan may be only to treat one tooth, or to have one procedure such as bleaching. Thus, patients have their own set of *desires*. You, however, may, and initially should, develop the *ideal* treatment plan. Realistically, the cost for the ideal plan may exceed the resources of the patient, and compromises may be necessary (Fig 10-3).

An excellent way to demonstrate to your patient that their initial desires may not be the best treatment plan is to use the *silent motivator*. Rather than presenting a picture of your ideal treatment plan or their desired plan, create a combination image of a before/desired/ideal treatment plan (Fig 10-4). Your patient can compare these three images side by side and select that which meets his or her esthetic requirements and financial restrictions. Because the patient can see that your ideal treatment plan offers the best results, he or she may not be able to resist it. This silent motivator image transforms you from a *seller* of dentistry to a *provider* of quality dentistry. And the patient becomes a well-informed, confident decision maker who is ready to proceed with treatment. And, most importantly, the possibility of esthetic failure or patient dissatisfaction is greatly reduced.

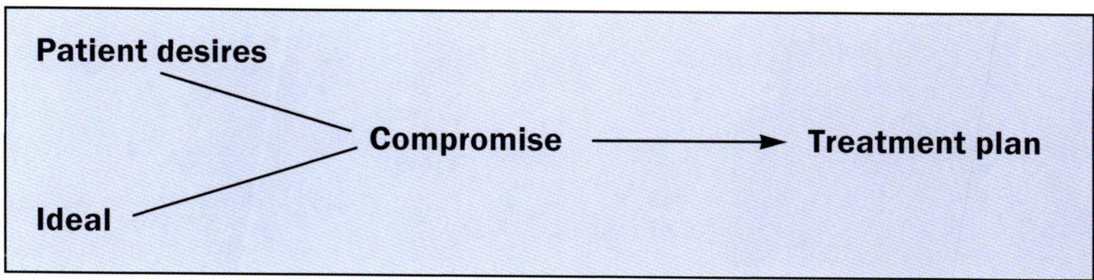

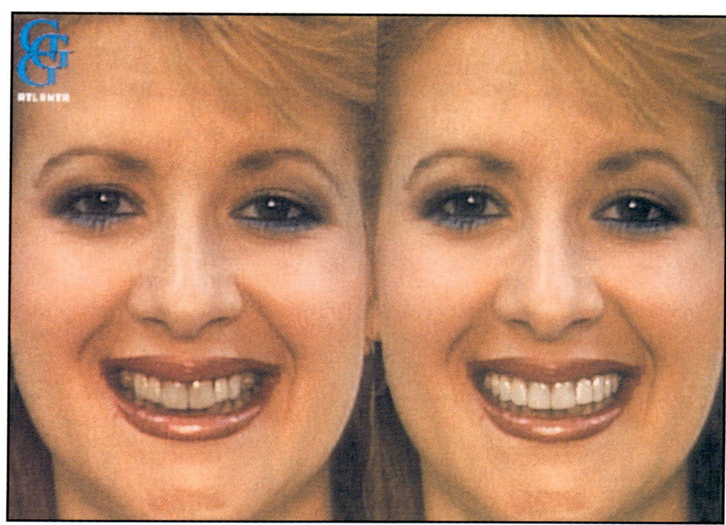

Fig 10-3 Left, The "before" image of a patient who wants six new laminates. Right, This image shows that the ideal treatment plan should be ten rather than her desired six laminates.

Fig 10-4 The silent motivator image places the patient's desired treatment plan next to your ideal plan (on the far right) for easy comparison.

Imaging and case presentation

Patient advantages	Doctor advantages
Easier to visualize, understand, and evaluate options	Accurate
A personalized treatment plan	Less misinterpretation
Patient becomes a co-diagnostician	Less "selling" needed
Can review at home, consult with family	Silent motivator
	Informed consent before treatment
	Reduced malpractice risk
	Increased treatment plan acceptance

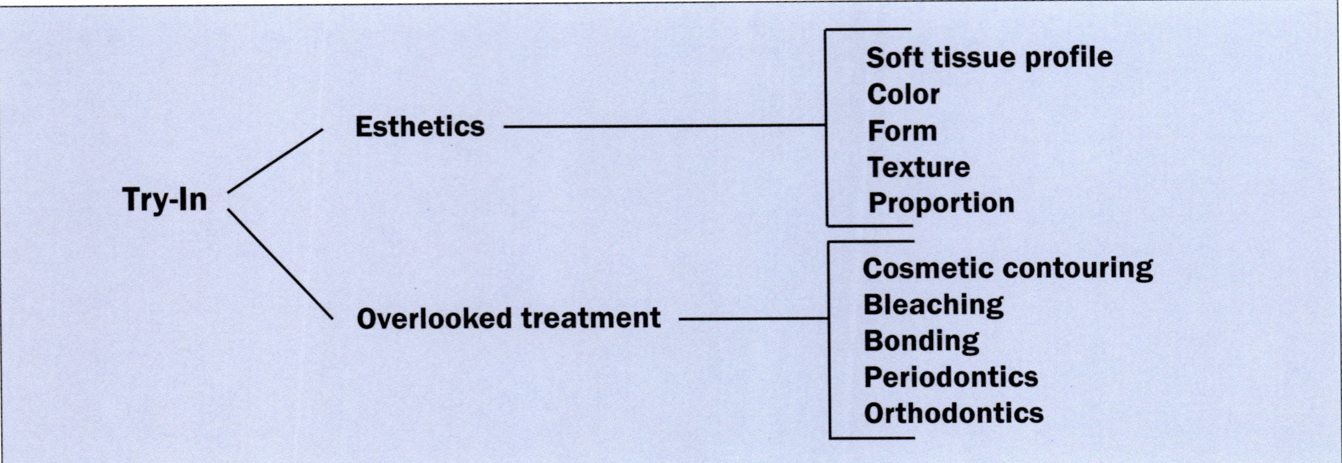

Try-in

The try-in phase is your final opportunity to validate that the restorations are perfect before they are glazed, polished, and cemented into your patient's mouth. Use close-up and smile images and the esthetic checklist to evaluate the condition of the restorations at this point and ensure that they are in line with the patient's original expectations. These try-in images can resolve any conflicts of esthetic interpretation between you and your patient while it is easy to correct the situation. For example, if you feel the restoration should be recontoured but your patient does not, proposed corrections first can be evaluated on the computer, and when and if agreed upon, performed on the restoration (Fig 10-5).

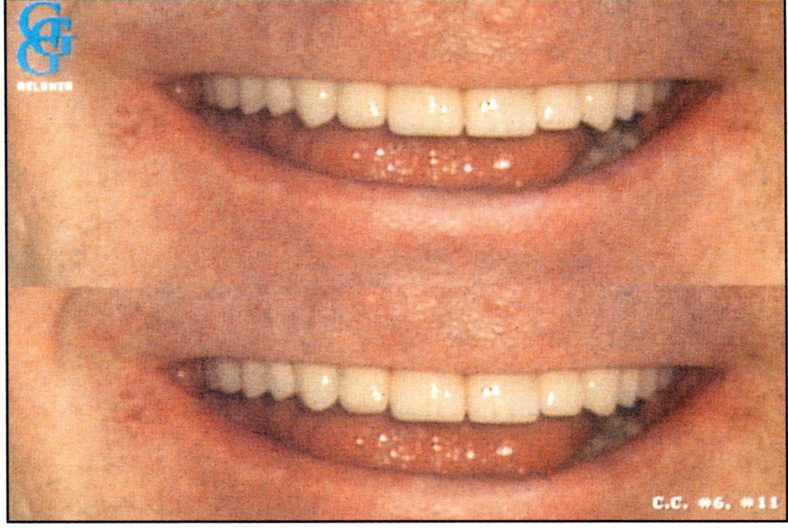

Fig 10-5 *Top, This man was pleased with his new crowns. Bottom, The cuspid tips have been subtly shortened and rounded for a more esthetic result.*

Try-In

Patient advantages	Doctor advantages
Allows patient to see in two dimensions	Saves time
Provides alternative views	Immediate correction
No surprises	Can detect overlooked treatment
	Resolves conflicts of esthetic interpretation

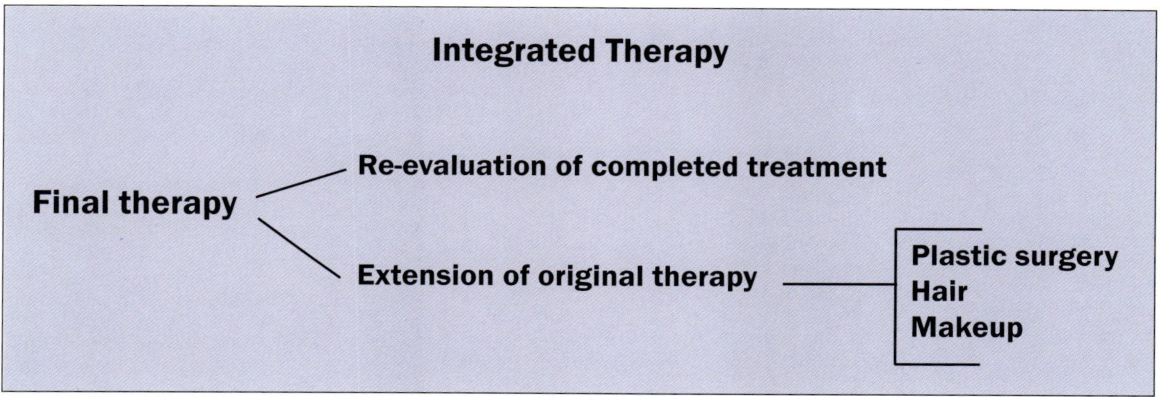

Final Therapy

This last phase of computer utilization allows you an opportunity to add further refinements that may guide the patient toward his or her full esthetic potential. Although you may have suggested integrated therapies during the diagnostic phase, now that the patient has his or her beautifully restored teeth and smile, this may be the perfect time to show how a new hairstyle or plastic surgery could enhance the new esthetic results (Fig 10-6a to c).

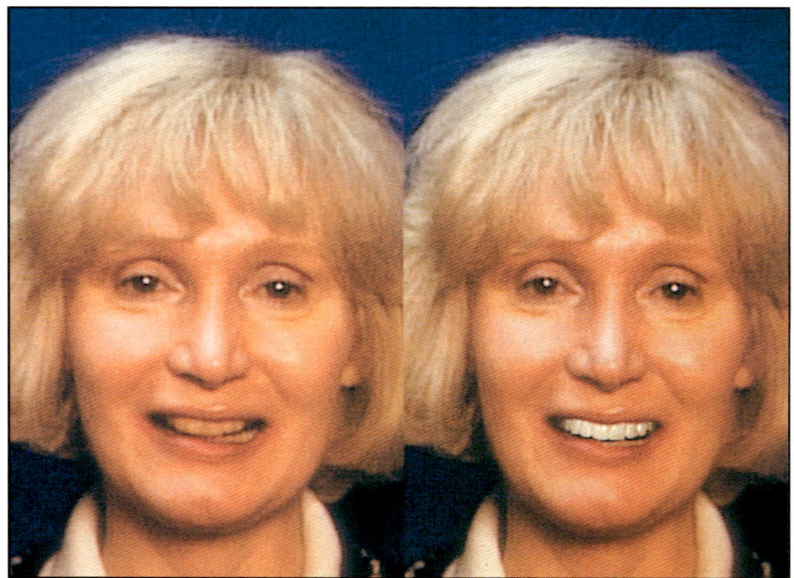

Fig 10-6a *Left. The patient's before photo. Right. The image of a patient with new crowns: the teeth are quite noticeable.*

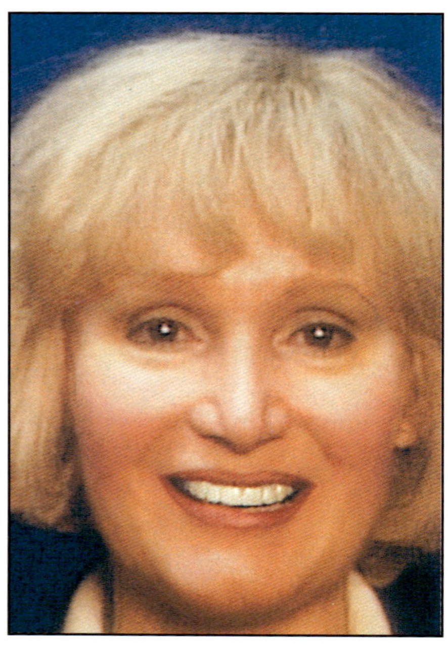

Fig 10-6b *Makeup has been applied, making the new teeth less conspicuous.*

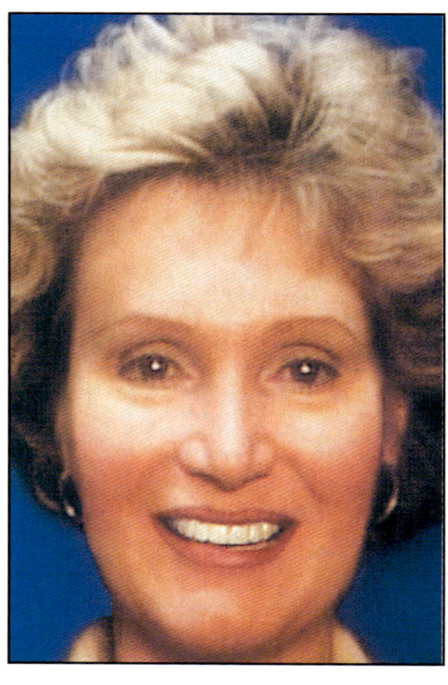

Fig 10-6c *Finally, the addition of a new hairstyle completes a total esthetic makeover for this patient.*

Integrated therapy

Patient advantages	**Doctor advantages**
Visualize new smile in relation to whole face	Improved esthetic results
Greater appreciation	Provides two-dimensional final analysis
Last chance for any minor changes	Possible extension of original therapy
	Last chance for minor changes

The *Finishing* Touches

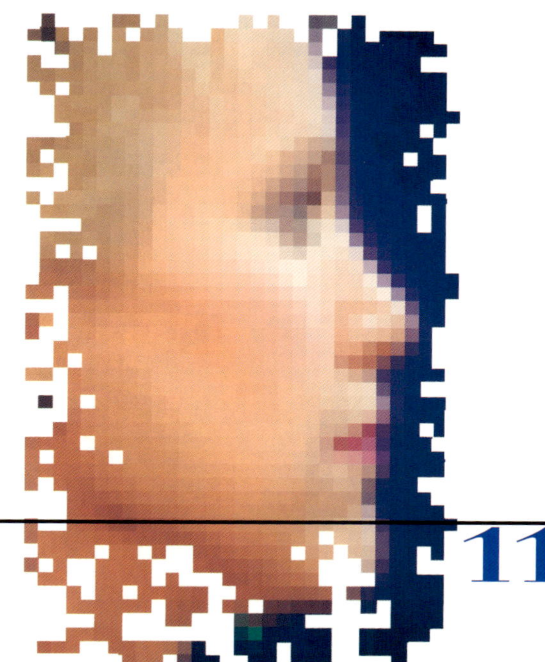

11

When patients come to you seeking esthetic improvement, they may be concerned with more than just their teeth; they may be considering other changes, such as orthognathic surgery or plastic surgery. In many cases, patients may want to improve their appearance without knowing precisely what is possible or how to go about it. You might ask the patient, "If you had a magic wand that would allow you to change anything about yourself, what would that change be?" This may prompt the patient to express personal dislikes about his or her appearance that would otherwise remain unknown to you.

A word of caution: regardless of your own response to the patient's esthetic appearance, tact and sensitivity on your part will serve you well. Listen carefully to the patient for comments or clues that might invite discussion of other esthetic changes, but do not impose your own esthetic sense unless clearly requested. You could find yourself helpfully suggesting rhinoplasty to someone who likes his or her distinctive nose. Needless to say, such a blunder is embarrassing. With a communicative and receptive patient, however, you are in an ideal position to use your esthetic imaging system to illustrate possible changes and then refer the patient to a plastic surgeon or oral surgeon.

Incorporating a plastic surgeon into your esthetic team not only offers more options to your patients, but extends your network of referrals. Moreover, a coordinated effort involving a plastic surgeon or craniofacial surgeon can often enhance your esthetic dentistry results. Because the results of such cooperation can be so beneficial for the patient, as well as you and your professional colleagues, we cannot overemphasize the value of establishing and maintaining meaningful referral relationships with other specialists. It is critical to inform each doctor in your referral network of each other's area of expertise and what realistically can be achieved within your areas of specialization. This will help to prevent inadvertently misleading a patient or raising false hopes about the scope or outcome of treatment.

The ideal approach is for you and the surgeon to meet jointly with the patient to discuss treatment options. However, if you work with plastic surgeons who have compatible computer systems, each doctor will be able to confer separately with the patient and then electronically exchange and build upon one another's esthetic imaging report.

The following are some broad guidelines for imaging minor esthetic changes that are beyond the scope of esthetic dentistry, but could be compatible with the esthetic goals of your patient.

Simulating Blepharoplasty

The eyes, second only to the smile as the most communicative part of a person's face, can have a dramatic impact on the overall esthetic image. Ptotic or drooping upper eyelids make a person look tired. Subcutaneous fat pads in the lower lids give a person a puffy-eyed appearance that also makes them look tired and old. Many people want to get rid of their wrinkles. Although it is easy to blend them away on the computer screen, be aware that it may be surgically impossible to remove wrinkles entirely. Some of those "crows feet" may still remain (Fig 11-1).

Many factors can affect surgical outcome. For example, if the patient is a smoker, the skin's ability to rebound is proportionately limited. With advancing age, the skin gradually loses its natural elasticity and corresponding ability to respond optimally to surgery. Also, there are cases when eyelid surgery will need to be combined with a coronoplasty, or "brow lift," to achieve optimum results.

To simulate surgery for correcting lines, puffiness, or bags under the eyes, use the blend brush (Fig 11-2, top left and right). If the under-eye area is dark, you may want to move some lighter color from the cheeks to the area before blending (Fig 11-2, bottom left and right). Use blend at its maximum setting.

There are two techniques for changing upper eyelids. The first works for minor changes (Fig 11-3).

1. Choose a dark brown or taupe color.
2. Recreate the new crease (lid) line with a curved line.
3. Darken the area from the new crease line to the brow with a taupe color.
4. Lighten the area underneath the new crease line if necessary.
5. Blend where lines and colors were added.

This will create the illusion of light hitting the new eyelid area, rather than under the brow, and will accent the eyes.

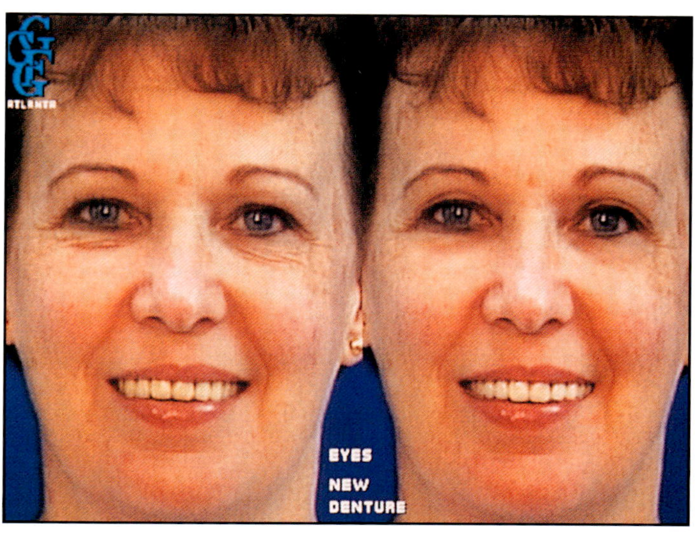

Fig 11-1 *Although you may be able to achieve perfection with your imaging simulations, remember that plastic surgery may not be able to match that perfection.*

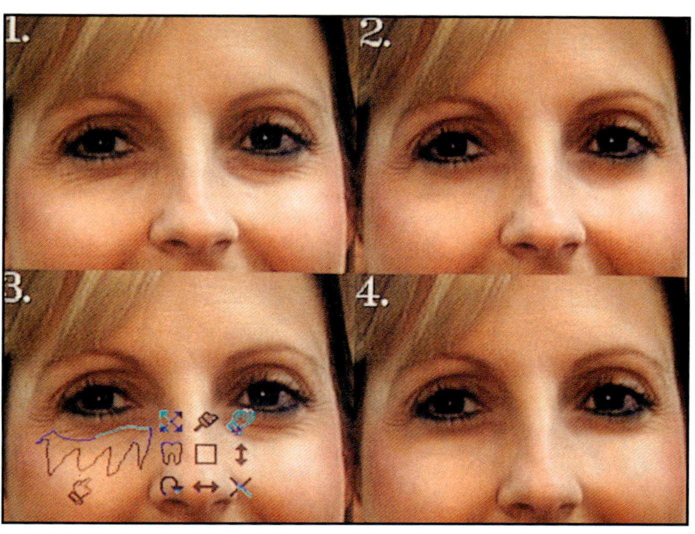

Fig 11-2 *The simplest way to correct puffiness under the eyes is to use the blend brush (upper left and right). If the area under the eyes becomes too dark, move a lighter color from the cheeks to the area under the eyes and blend (lower left and right).*

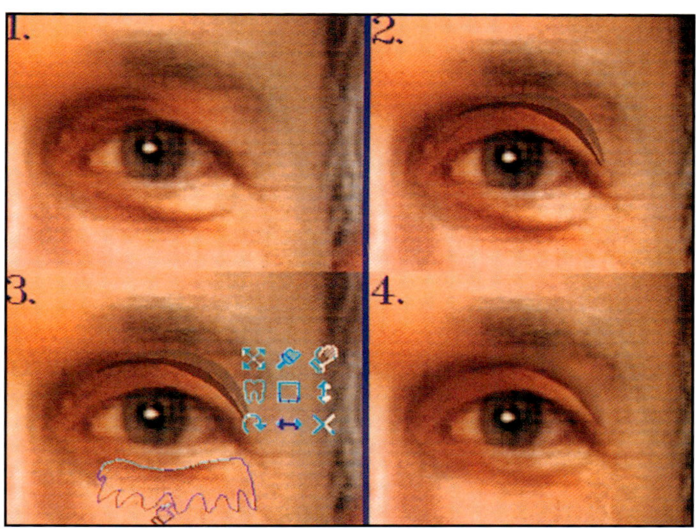

Fig 11-3 *Upper left, Before the eyelid change. Upper right, The dark line creates the new lid line, and the lighter taupe color darkens the area just above the crease. Lower left, The area under the eye is lightened. Lower right, All areas are blended for a smooth appearance.*

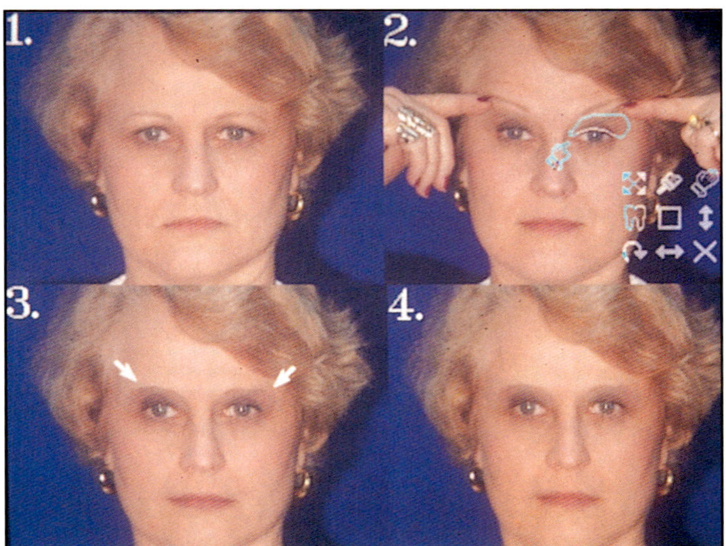

Fig 11-4 Upper left. The normal full-face image. Upper right. A second image is captured with the patient elevating her eyebrows. Lower left. Replace the eyes from step 1 with those from step 2. Lower right. Use the blend function to achieve a final result.

The second technique can improve the appearance of drooping upper eyelids that obscure part of the eye:

1. Capture a normal full-face image (Fig 11-4, top left).
2. Capture a second image with the patient elevating the brows using the hands (Fig 11-4, top right).
   - Be sure the head position is the same as in the first picture.
   - The patient should not open their eyes too widely for this raised brow image. (The hands will not be visible in the final result.)
3. Beginning with the second image, save windows of both eyes.
4. Replace the original droopy lidded eyes with the windows of the open ones (Fig 11-4, bottom left).
5. Use the copy or erase function to restore the portions of the original image you want to save (Fig 11-4, bottom right).
6. Use the maximum blend to finish.

Simulating Rhinoplasty

The nose is usually the anterior-most projection of the face, and with its mid-point positioning, it is the major esthetic mass of the face.[1] Minor alterations to the nose dimensions may result in more harmony or balance to the entire face. For imaging most changes in the nose, the profile image is usually best (Fig 11-5).

For specific changes within the nose, start with the profile image (Fig 11-6a, left).

1. If indicated, rotate the tip of the nose up (Fig 11-6a, middle).
2. You may also move the tip of the nose forward or back (Fig 11-6a, right).
3. Generally the columella–lip angle should be:
   - 90 degrees in a man
   - Between 105 and 110 degrees in a woman (Fig 11-6b, left)
   - In younger patients, a larger angle is required; this angle will usually be reduced as the patient ages.
   - Be aware that most noses tend to droop with age.
4. Using the background color, reshape the nose profile from bridge to tip (Fig 11-6, middle and right).

Fig 11-5 *The lateral full-face view is best for evaluating nasal changes.*

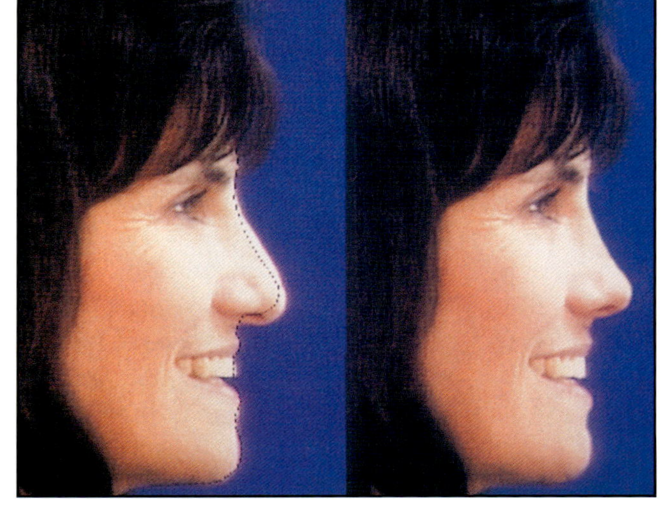

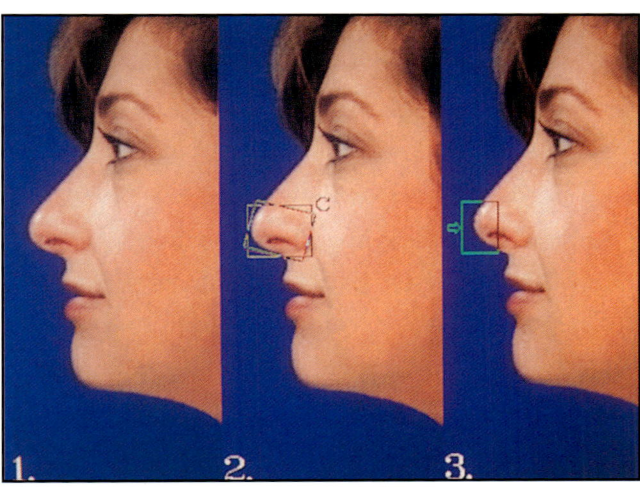

Fig 11-6a *Left, The profile "before" image. Middle, The tip is rotated upwards. Right, The tip is repositioned towards the face.*

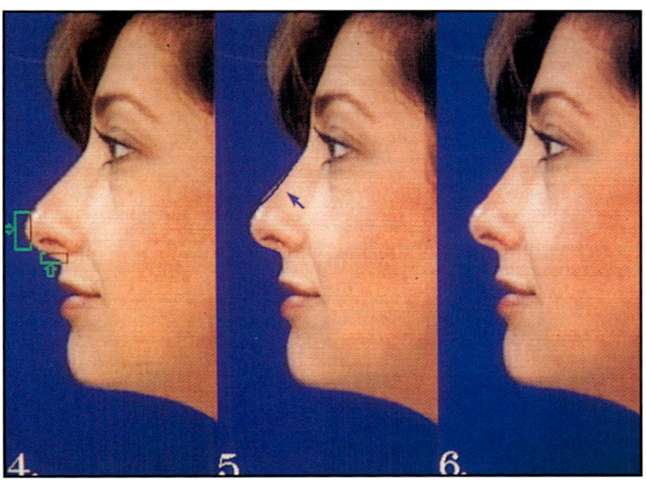

Fig 11-6b *Left, The columella–lip angle is between 105 and 110 degrees in women. Middle, The bridge to the tip is reshaped. Right, All changes are blended.*

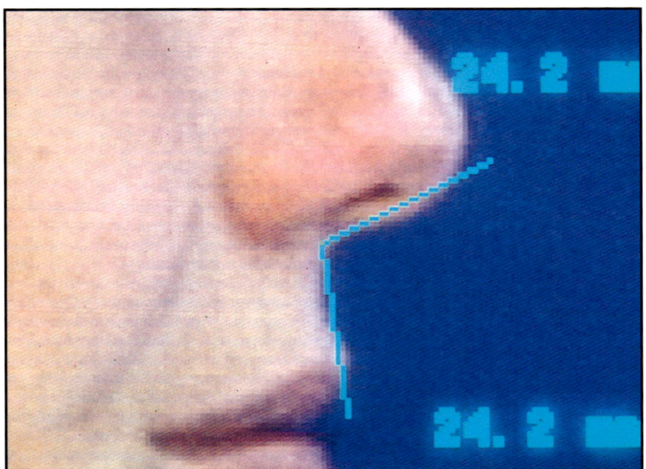

Fig 11-7 Notice the 1:1 ratio of the projection of the nose to the length of the upper lip.

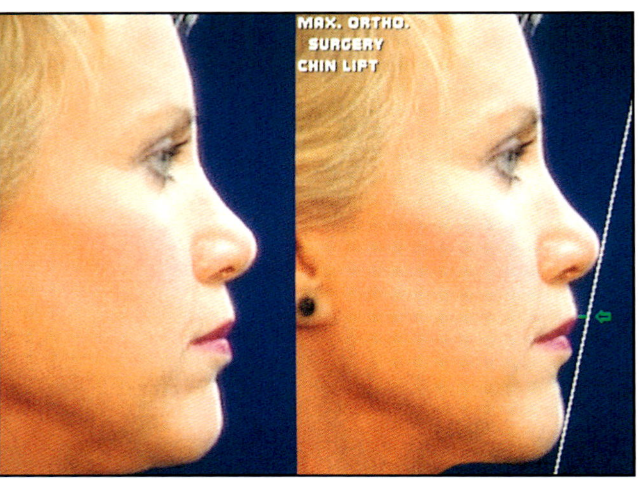

Fig 11-8 A space of approximately 2 mm should exist from the edge of the upper lip to a line drawn from the tip of the nose to the tip of the chin.

5. The angle at the bridge of the nose should occur near the eyelashes.
6. The line of the nose usually breaks a little above the tip, especially in women. Men's noses tend to be straighter.
7. The usual ratio between the distance the nose projects from the face and the length of the upper lip is 1:1 (Fig 11-7).
8. A line drawn from the tip of the chin to the tip of the nose should extend about 2 mm from the upper lip (Fig 11-8).

Simulating Mentoplasty or Mandibular Resection

The chin should help balance the rest of the face. Any change to the chin may change the lower lip posture and will either flatten or deepen the mentolabial sulcus. Chins, like noses, are usually best analyzed and modified from a profile aspect. An image of the patient's cephalometric radiograph can be captured showing plotted movements and measurements. Sections can then be moved to show how hard and soft tissue will relate (Fig 11-9).

Some patients may think they need their nose shortened when a better alternative is to move the chin forward. Computer imaging can help your patients understand the different approaches and perhaps keep them from making a change that might be to their esthetic disadvantage, which, in this case, might make the face appear too flat.

To show changes in chin position:

1. Move the chin forward or back.
2. Blend or reshape with the background color to create smooth changes in the chin line (Fig 11-10a).
3. You can also show how submental lipoplasty, or fat suctioning under the chin, can make a dramatic difference in the patient's profile.
4. To reshape the neck, use a curving line and the background color (Fig 11-10b).

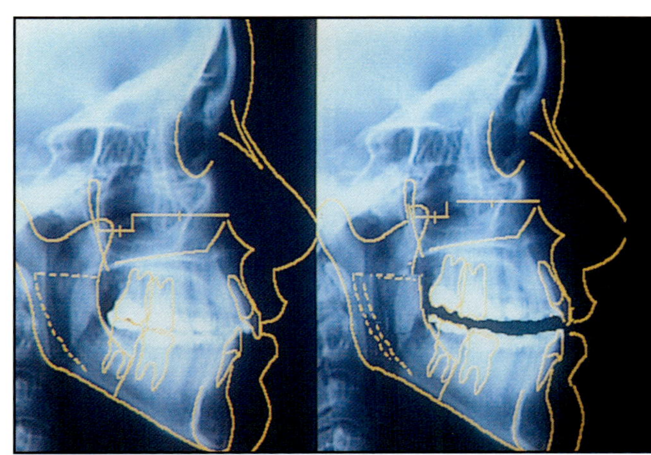

Fig 11-9 *Chin movement can be plotted and moved cephalometrically.*

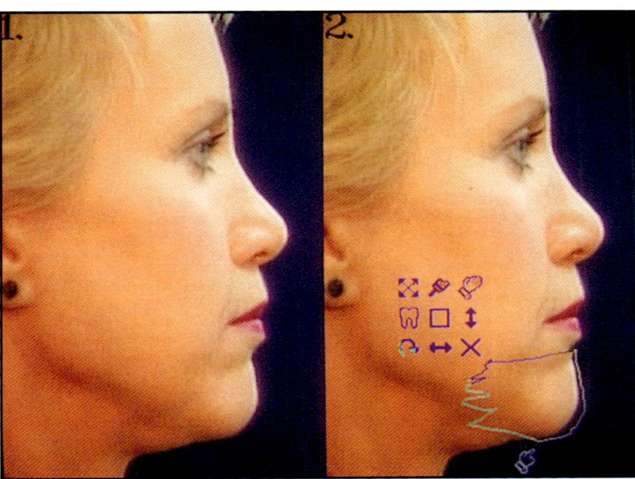

Fig 11-10a *The chin is easily moved back or forward with a framed move.*

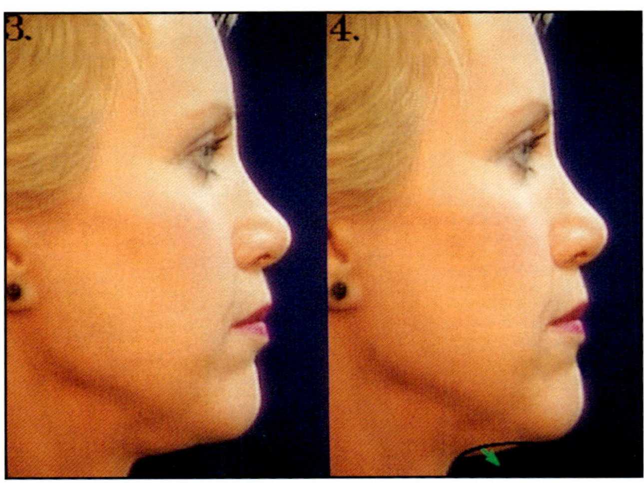

Fig 11-10b *Use the background color to remove a double chin.*

Simulating Dermabrasion or Chemical Peel

Dermabrasion, laser resurfacing, and chemical peels are procedures that remove the top layer of skin and reduce or eliminate many of the wrinkles that come with age, as well as for cases of severe acne scarring. Dermabrasion is a mechanical procedure using a fine wire brush, or similar instrument, to abrade the skin; a chemical peel uses a mild acid to burn the top skin layer. While the immediate post-treatment results are not very attractive, the final results can be highly satisfactory. The patient should avoid any prolonged exposure to direct sunlight after treatment indefinitely. Both procedures are popular and their effects can be illustrated on the computer by blending the affected area until the skin appears smooth (Fig 11-11). Use the blend brush at its maximum setting.

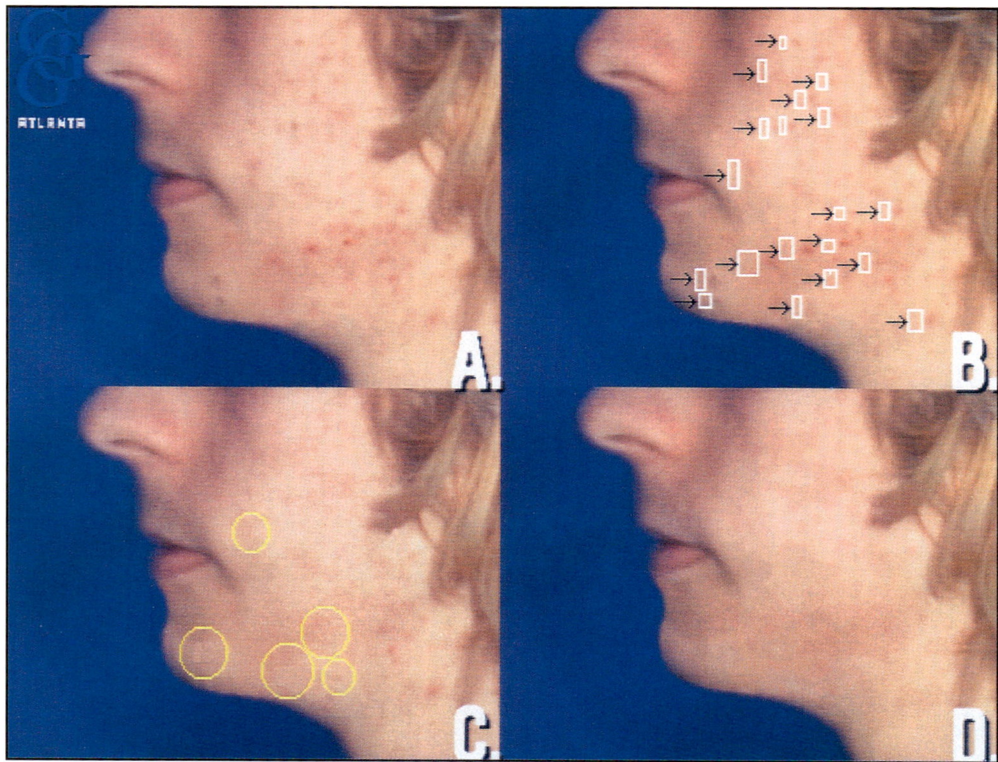

Fig 11-11 Dermabrasion is one of the easiest plastic surgery procedures to simulate—simply use the blend tool.

Simulating Liposuction

Because the results of lipoplasty vary for each patient, this imaging procedure should be performed by the plastic surgeon. However, some minor changes can be imaged if you have some basic guidance from your referring plastic surgeon.

Cosmetic Flourishes

The addition of color or simple shadowing to certain areas of the face, or a change of hairstyle, can enhance a patient's appearance. These changes can be the special touch that make esthetic dental treatment all the more successful and appreciated by your patients, their families, and friends.

Your goal for computerized makeup imaging is to enhance your patient's better features and to de-emphasize others.

It is essential to understand how to use makeup and hairstyles before you offer this service option. There are many courses and written guides that explain how to achieve remarkable results with cosmetology. You may purchase a computerized hair bank, or create one yourself to simplify changing your patient's hairstyle, color, or cut on the computer (Fig 11-12a to c; see also p. 87).

Finally, note how the shape of the face can be modified by altering the hairstyle. For example, a square or wide face can appear more round or slender with a different hairstyle. Longer hair tends to make the face appear thinner or more oval, and conversely short hair can widen a thin face. Hair color often is a matter of personal preference. Because hair color affects the overall appearance of the face, patients should be advised to select a natural-appearing color that complements the skin tones (Fig 11-12b and c).

Makeup

Artfully applied makeup can achieve remarkable results. Your goal for computerized make-up imaging is to enhance your patient's better features and to de-emphasize others. Begin by looking at the image of the face as a whole. Facial proportion can be made to appear more harmonious by emphasizing deficient areas with washes of lighter color and diminishing prominent ones with darker shading.

1. Brown or taupe washes, used under cheek bones, the chin, or at the temple, can create the illusion of a perfectly oval face (Fig 11-13).
2. Wide noses can be narrowed with similar contouring (Fig 11-14).

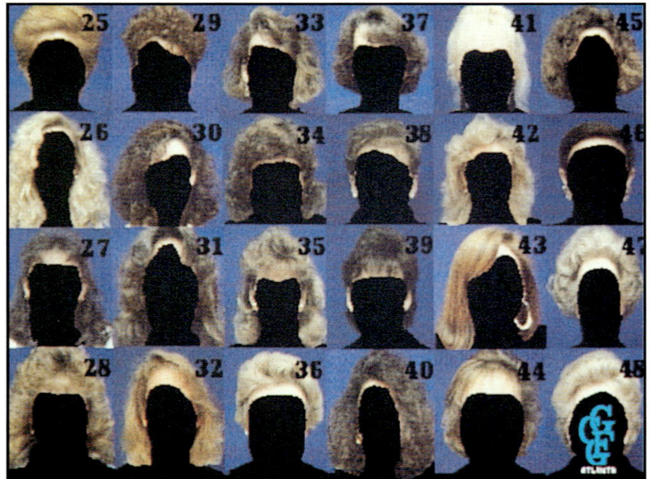

Fig 11-12a *A hair bank allows you to view numerous hairstyles quickly.*

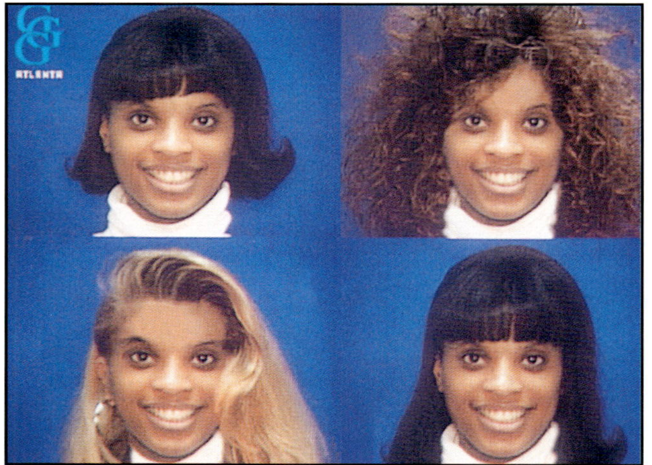

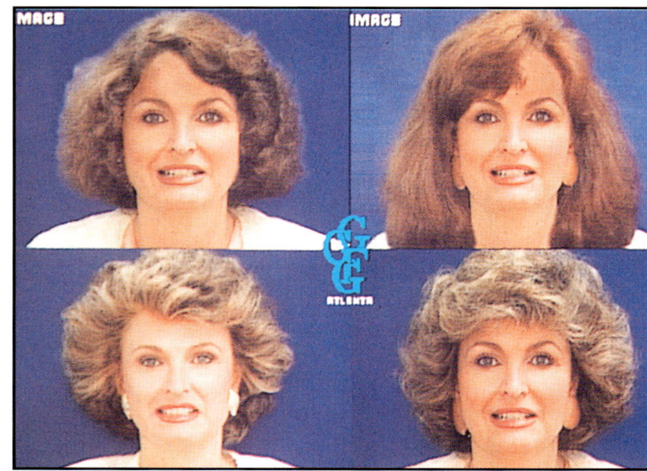

Fig 11-12b and c *Notice how different hairstyles and colors change facial shape and overall appearance.*

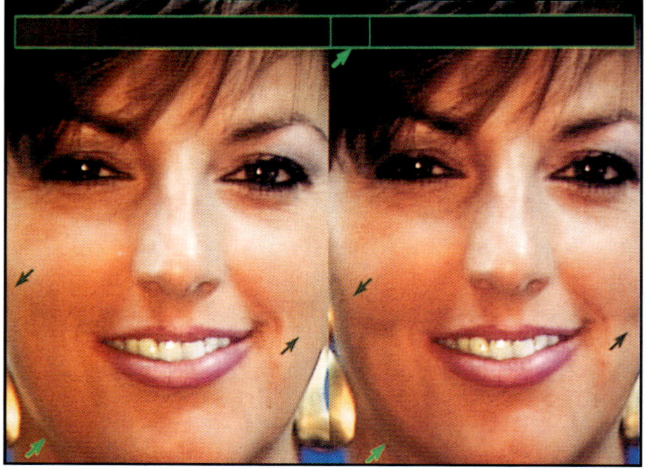

Fig 11-13 *Placing washes of color in the indicated areas helps to create the illusion of an oval face.*

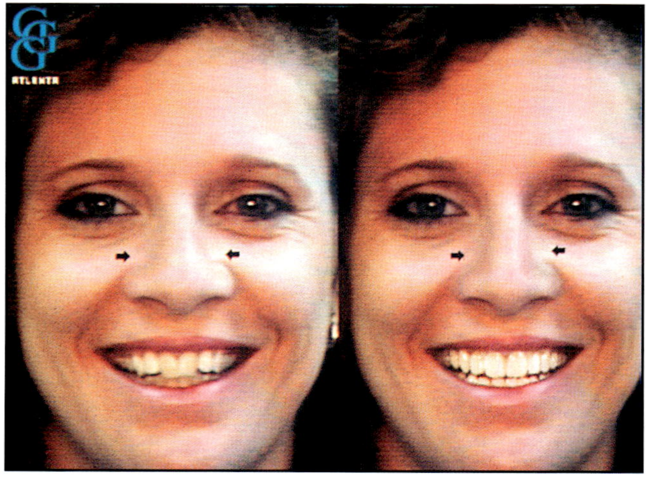

Fig 11-14 *The nose can be contoured with washes of color to make it appear smaller.*

3. Color washes can be lifted from the image itself or selected from the imaging system's color bar.
4. Save the image after each progressive change to eliminate starting over if you create something unsatisfactory in an intermediate step.

Eyes. The eyes are one of the main focal points of the face. Proper highlighting of the eyes can enhance your patient's overall appearance.

Ideal eyebrow shape can be determined with simple guidelines:

1. A vertical line extending from beside the nostril to the forehead will indicate where the brow should begin, unless the nose is overly broad (Fig 11-15, left).
2. A line extending from beside the nostril to the outside of the eye determines brow length (Fig 11-15, right).
3. The arch of the brow normally occurs immediately above the center of the pupil when the patient is looking straight ahead.

To make eyes appear larger:

1. Use taupe or brown washes on the area between the brow and the lid. Angle the color slightly upward toward the outside (Fig 11-16, top left and right).
2. Apply lighter color to the eyelid (Fig 11-16, bottom left).
3. Gently blend to remove any sharp delineations between the colors (Fig 11-16, bottom right).

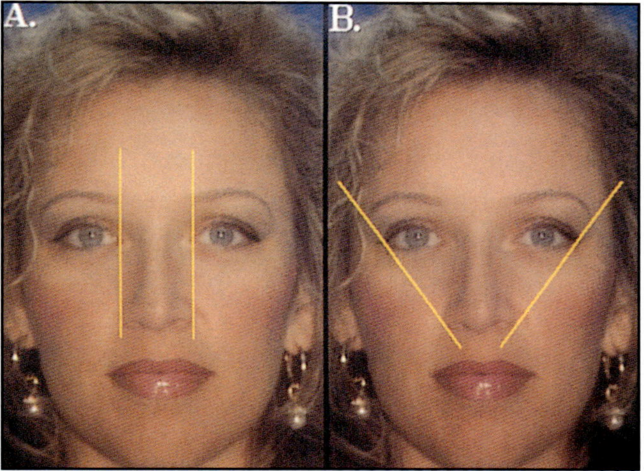

Fig 11-15a and b *Eyebrow length can be determined by these sets of lines.*

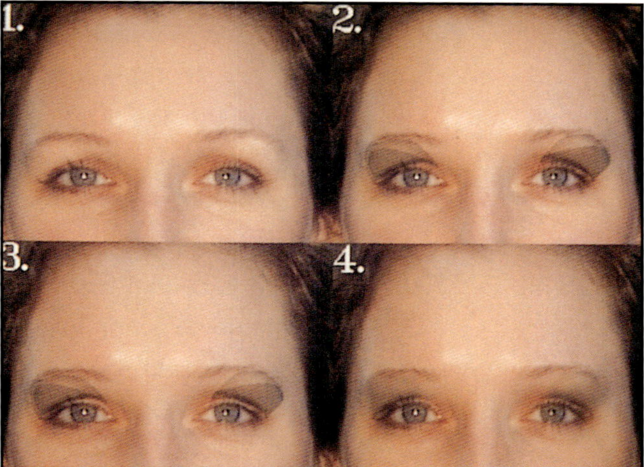

Fig 11-16 *Upper left, The before image of the patient. Upper right, Washes of color are applied to the eyelid area and angled upwards. Lower left, Lighter color is placed just over the eye. Lower right, All these washes are blended to create an illusion of larger eyes.*

To help separate close-set eyes:

Lighten the area between the eye and the bridge of the nose.

Cheeks. Makeup artists often apply blush in three dots of color and blend them in a comma shape to accentuate the cheek bones (Fig 11-17)

1. The first dot goes under the eye on the apple of the cheek (Fig 11-17, top right).
2. The second dot is placed back and somewhat lower, but still above the nostril level.
3. The third dot is placed back and up toward the ear.
4. Gently blend these dots of color (Fig 11-17, bottom left and right).

Lips. The lips are the framework for the mouth and often the focal point of the face. Proper contouring and color of the lips will accentuate and flatter your imaged esthetic dental changes. Because most imaged new restorations will be in the Vita A-1 to B-1 range, the teeth may appear truly white on the computer.

Remember, the computer shows relative color, making it a tool for comparison rather than accuracy.

Bright reds added to the lips tend to make the teeth appear whiter. Remember, the computer shows *relative* color, making it a tool for comparison rather than accuracy. Imaging can play an important role when you and your patient are making the critical decision between a natural-appearing tooth color or one that is brighter. For example, if your patient feels that the imaged teeth are too bright, you can manipulate the color of the teeth, the lips, or both, to a more subtle tone. The ability to see and agree on color issues and accurately communicate the decisions to the laboratory technician is an important advantage to everyone.

To apply color to the lips, first outline them with a shade slightly darker than the actual lip color (Fig 11-18).

Makeup can be considered another accessory in the wardrobe. Brightly colored clothes require bright makeup, while subtle colors call for more restrained makeup. In either case, makeup shades can be picked up from clothing. Excellent cosmetology books are available if you wish to learn more about shade selection to complement a person's natural coloring.

Tips:

- Dark colors appear to diminish features.
- Light colors appear to advance and expand features.
- Use color sparingly for a natural look.
- Lines should angle up and back for a youthful look.
- Blend colors carefully after contouring.

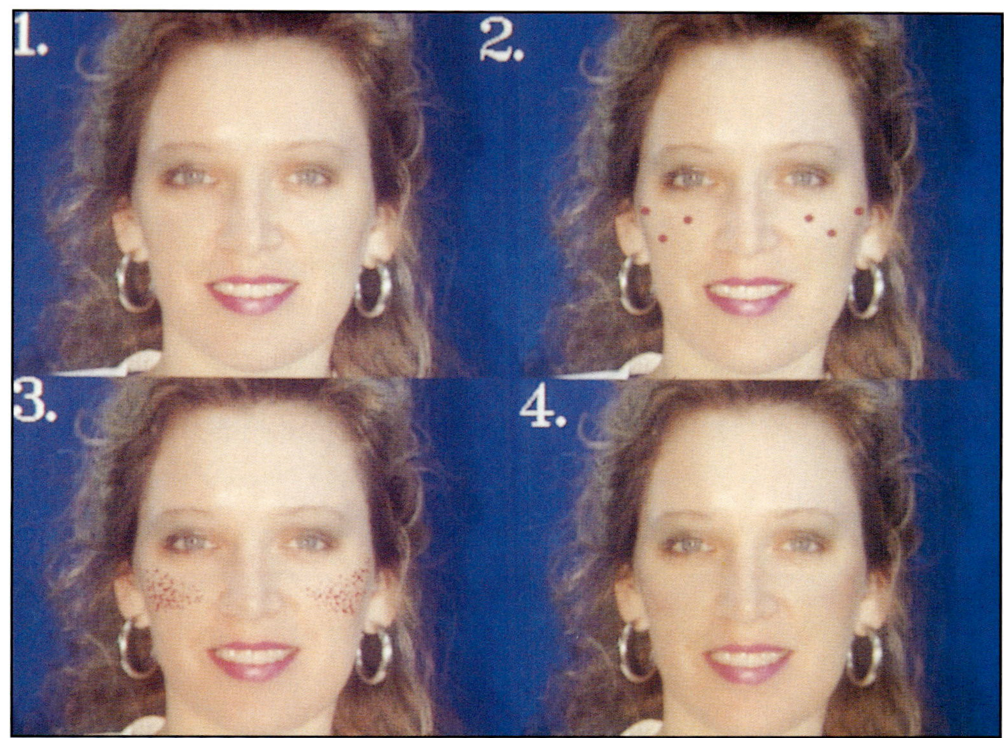

Fig 11-17 Adding color to the cheeks gives the illusion of more prominent cheek bones.

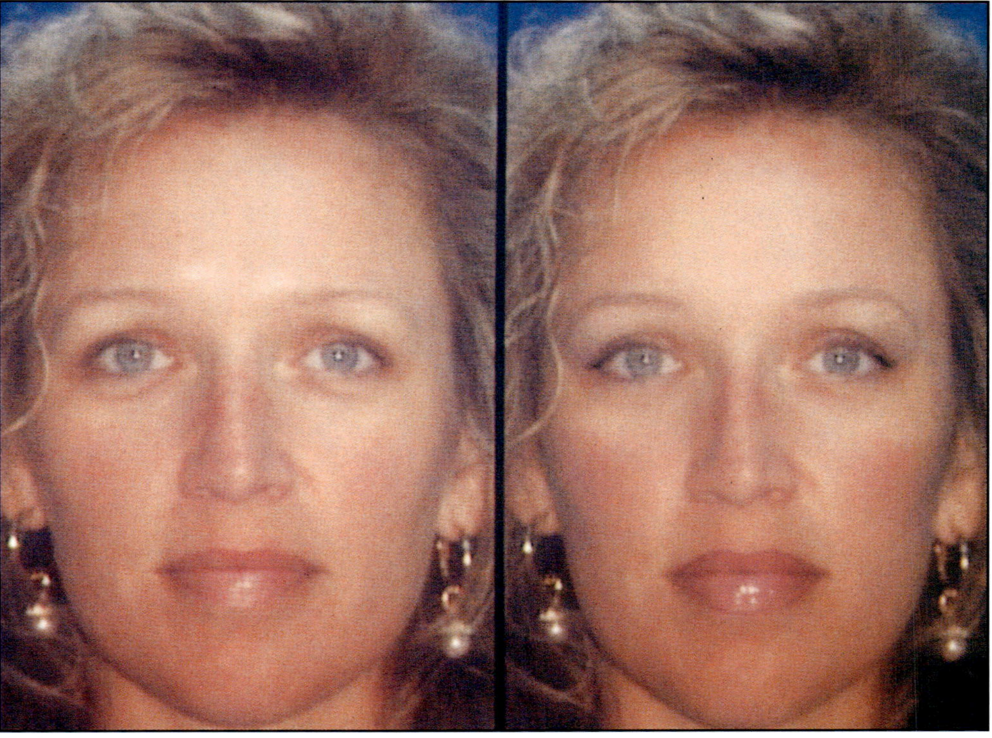

Fig 11-18 When applying lip color, first outline the lips with a color that is a shade darker than the color used on the lips themselves.

Combination Therapy

This integrated approach may involve any of the disciplines that have been discussed. Through the use of the computerized image, patients can see how each proposed discipline can affect their goal for an esthetic makeover (Fig 11-19a and b). Further, they can determine if modifying or eliminating any aspect will cause them to be dissatisfied with the long-term results of their therapy. Imaging provides a pictorial blueprint to logically plan for complicated treatments involving more than one discipline and/or specialist.[2] And it gives the dentist the ability to present the array of available esthetic options to the patient in a clear and highly personalized format.

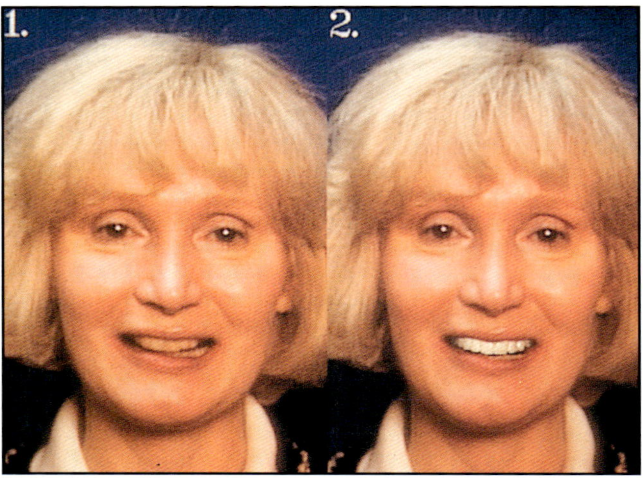

Fig 11-19a *Left, The "before" image. Right, The projected image with a new smile.*

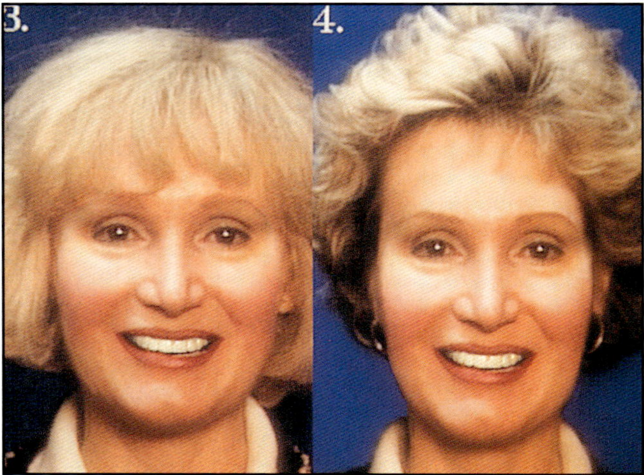

Fig 11-19b *Left, Notice how the addition of makeup changes the face. Right, A new hairstyle is added to show how each of the beauty concepts is used to achieve an esthetic result.*

References

1. Powell N, Humphreys B. Proportions of the Esthetic Face. New York: Thieme-Stratton, 1984:20.
2. VanderKam VM, Achaner BM. Digital imaging for plastic and reconstructive surgery. Plast Surg Nurs 1997;17:37–38.

Integrating Imaging into Your Practice

12

Arlen Lackey, DDS

Having read this far, you now have a good idea of the potential benefits computer imaging can bring to your practice, including improved dentist-patient communication, enhanced treatment planning, improved communication with the laboratory, improved staff understanding, improved case documentation, and practice building.[1,2,3]

Imaging Costs and Income Production

While a computer imaging system offers many advantages, it is a significant investment for most dental practices and one that should be weighed carefully.

While a computer imaging system offers many advantages, it is a significant investment for most dental practices and one that should be weighed carefully. Before you can make an informed decision, you should consider three main issues of an imaging system: acquisition cost, space, and staffing.[4]

The capital outlay of an imaging system can be offset by its potential as an additional income base. The following statistics can help you rationalize the cost: A U.S. growth-oriented solo general practice may see 16 to 22 new patients a month. If half are imaged, assuming an average charge of $45 for the service, 10 new patients will generate $450 of income. In addition, the office continuing-care or recare program may contribute an additional two to three patients weekly for imaging consultation. Eight hygiene patient consultations at $45 each adds $360 monthly. Of these 18 imaged patients, perhaps 25 percent (one out of four) will expand their treatment plan by a unit or two of crowns or veneers ($500 to $900) and add, as an extremely conservative average, $2,400 of production. Let's total these estimates:

Fees for imaging new patients	$450
Fees for imaging recall patients	$360
Treatment expansion	$2,400
Total Monthly Income	$3,210

This estimate of the additional income that can be generated monthly by imaging illustrates the potential for imaging equipment to pay for itself, establish a new profit center and, most importantly, enable you to provide expanded health services for your patients.[5]

How Much Should You Spend?

Multiplying the previously estimated $3,210 by six successful months amounts to $19,260, a sum sufficient to purchase a system outright. However, a rental or lease arrangement may be a more attractive alternative for technology acquisitions. Today, most offices acquire or upgrade to Windows-based software systems knowing that there are options available for integrated imaging software. These options carry an approximate cost of $4,000 to $6,000 and include a portable digital camera. Regardless of the financial approach you take to acquiring an imaging system, if you make the effort to fully integrate the imaging services into your practice, the true cost of ownership will be negligible because of the return on investment potential.

How Much Should You Charge?

Equipment purchases or lease costs, maintenance, and operational costs (including labor and training) must all be factored in when determining the fees for imaging services, along with the amount of time necessary to image the patient. For uncomplicated cases with patients well prepared for the consultation, fees would likely be lower than those for patients who have many questions or ask to expand the typical imaging session with options such as wrinkle removal, a new hair style, or other cosmetic changes.

Fees sampled across the U.S. for new-patient imaging consultations range from zero to $250, with the average fee ranging from $45 to $95. Offices charging the higher amount will often credit some or all of the imaging fee toward the treatment plan, thus encouraging treatment plan acceptance. Fees for imaging recare patients are similar to above, although the average is lowered to about $45 to $65.

An alternative approach is to include imaging at no charge for both initial consultations and recare patients. The rationale is to image as many patients as possible, relying on the technology's power to motivate patients to pursue esthetic or functional improvements. When you charge for imaging, many patients may consider it an unnecessary frill or expense and reject it outright. But given a no-cost, no-risk opportunity to see and evaluate what can be accomplished for them with modern dental techniques, many patients will adopt at least part of the ensuing treatment plan. Thus, an imaging system can become an integral part of building your practice.

Making Room for an Imaging System

Acquiring a computer imaging system is just the first step in incorporating this technology in your practice. The next step is determining the best location for the equipment and for conducting the imaging consultations with patients.

Extraoral imaging can be done in any treatment room, but the trend among clinicians is to create a dedicated imaging consultation room—a comfortable setting with a pleasing decor designed not only to obtain the best-quality images, but to put patients at ease so they feel free to discuss their needs, wants, and expectations. (This concept applies only to extraoral imaging; intraoral imaging should be done in a treatment room.) With rising costs of office space, at first it may seem ill-advised to devote precious square footage to a dedicated consultation area. But this area can become some of your most productive space. It will enable you to clearly demonstrate to your patients—in privacy and without distractions—the benefits and value of the dental treatment options you can offer them.

Extraoral imaging can be done in any treatment room, but the trend among clinicians is to create a dedicated imaging consultation room.

When selecting the space for your imaging system, be sure the room is free of anything that might cause electrical interference with the computer equipment, such as large electrical panels and circuit boards. The space also must be large enough to obtain full-face views of the patient as well as close-ups. Since most video cameras have zoom capabilities, this is usually not a problem.

Choosing an Imaging Technician

The question of who in your practice is the best person to perform imaging services is an involved one. With today's user-friendly equipment and software, most anyone with one or two hours of training can learn the basics of computer imaging; little or no previous computer experience is necessary. Some type of training is normally included in the cost of an imaging system. Along with a training manual and user documentation, most software packages feature on-screen prompts to help users learn the system. Verify in your contract the training and documentation that is provided by your vendor.

Before you can decide who will assume the role of imaging technician, consider these questions: First, who has the required knowledge and skills or the ability to acquire them? Then, who among them has the time and interest?

What skills are necessary to maximize your imaging system investment? Naturally, to competently render the results of various procedures, an imaging technician should have a good understanding of dental treatment modalities and the related technical issues. Formal art training, while it may be desirable, is probably not required. But a good eye for details, such as the proper placement of highlights and shadows, will yield more effective, lifelike images that will aid patient understanding of treatment goals.

The imaging technician must also be able to communicate well with patients. Ideally, he or she should be able to listen with sensitivity and interpret the patient reactions to treatment alternatives. Likewise, an ability to explain treatment proposals and limitations in necessary detail and in layperson's terms is essential.

An imaging technician should have a good understanding of dental treatment modalities and the related technical issues. Formal art training, while it may be desirable, is probably not required.

As the dentist, you may already have decided that you are best qualified to do the imaging, and that may be best for you. However, if you intend to base your fees for this service on your normal hourly rate, you will probably price the service out of range of acceptance for most of your patients. On the other hand, imaging may be a procedure you would enjoy doing, in which case the amount of the fee may be secondary. Ultimately, you may find yourself with expanded treatment cases while at the same time you improve the quality of care and patient satisfaction, negating your initial intent to charge a fee at all.

Disregarding fees for a moment, do you have the time to take on an additional role? Although many plastic surgeons do their own facial profile changes, altering the smile may take a great deal longer than changing the angle of a patient's nose. A second option is to identify a staff member who not only has the appropriate dental background and an artistic eye, but who would also find the added job dimension intellectually stimulating. It's safe to assume that a staff person's time could be charged out at a lesser rate than yours. In a solo practice, the chairside dental assistant might be trained as an imaging technician; larger group practices offer a wider opportunity to cross train multiple staff members on the imaging system.[6]

Another option is to hire a part- or full-time computer imaging technician who has the appropriate dental and artistic background for the job. Such a person might also assume additional office or therapy responsibilities in your practice. Some larger cosmetic dental offices employ a dental hygienist who possesses the excellent communication skills required for this position.

Imaging as a Marketing Aid

An imaging system can be leveraged in many ways to help market your practice. For example, you can purchase a color thermal printer for your imaging system, enabling patients to leave your office with a picture of their intended treatment results in hand. In many instances, they will show this picture, which has your name or logo on it, to families, friends, or coworkers. More importantly, your patients will convey an entirely new dimension of dentistry to their individual circles of influence. They may encourage friends and family to try this new approach to dental treatment at your office.

This internal marketing by satisfied patients is the most effective and affordable form of marketing available. When you inform your existing and dormant patient population of your new computer-imaging technology service, you could stimulate and sustain the growth of your practice for many years.

Another marketing approach is to develop demonstration sessions or form a local study group to share ideas and information about this new technology with other dentists in your area. Interested practitioners may wish to have your office assist them in arranging imaging workups of their selected patients. Suitable fee arrangements can be worked out for all concerned.

Integrated therapy study clubs involving an orthodontist, orthognathic surgeon, plastic surgeon, periodontist, or other specialists usually use slides to discuss a patient's treatment plan. With a computer imaging system, you can make changes while the group observes. Not only is this more effective than static slides, it also makes it possible for each specialist to contribute their perspective and allows the group to consider and determine the most appropriate course of treatment. For example, lengthy orthodontic treatment might be ruled out if orthognathic surgery can achieve the same or better results in a shorter period of time.

External marketing can be directed toward local radio and television talk shows. Many of these shows feature innovative solutions to typical patient concerns and problems; high-tech dental advances make "good copy" in this environment. A few exploratory phone calls and a willingness to be adventurous can successfully add a new dimension to your practice-building efforts.

Local business and service clubs are often interested in topics such as advances in cosmetic dentistry. You or an appropriate member of your staff can make presentations featuring your imaging services and the dental treatments you like and perform best. To make your presentation even more attractive and further enhance your practice promotion, hold a drawing for a free computer imaging session at your office.

Before implementing your imaging services and/or the associated marketing activities, be sure to devise a method for measuring the effects that they will have on your practice.

You may wish to take a less entrepreneurial approach and focus on building outside patient referrals from your network of health-care and service professionals. These can be categorized into three principal groups: dental specialists such as oral surgeons and periodontists; medical specialists such as plastic surgeons and otorhinolaryngologists; and cosmetologists and hair stylists. Any of these professionals may be interested in helping a patient who wants to optimize his or her appearance. You can help create awareness of your services by giving complimentary copies of *Change Your Smile*[1] to your contacts. Inscribe such books with a personal salutation and attach your business card.

In summary, develop your marketing activities with careful attention to strategy and details. Equally important, incorporate only those activities with which you are comfortable and which are comfortable with your value system. Before implementing your imaging services and/or the associated marketing activities, be sure to devise a method for measuring the effects that they will have on your practice. Today's emerging technologies are being molded into seamless, fully integrated systems that will help practitioners reach new heights for quality of care and excellence of service in dentistry.[7,8]

References

1. Goldstein RE. Change Your Smile, ed 3. Chicago: Quintessence, 1997.
2. Garber DA, Goldstein RE, Feinman RA. Porcelain Laminate Veneers. Chicago: Quintessence, 1988.
3. Goldstein RE, Garber DA. Complete Dental Bleaching. Chicago: Quintessence, 1995.
4. Lackey AD. Examining your smile. Dent Clin North Am 1989;33:133.
5. Lackey AD. Computer imaging provides improved presentations. Dental Economics 1988;77:25–30.
6. Lackey AD. Personnel management: keeping the dental team together. J Am Dent Assoc 1987;114:772–779.
7. Lackey AD. New information base: integrated and networked computers. Calif Dental Assoc J 1994;22:18–22.
8. Lackey AD. Treatment room computers: enhancing scheduling, examination and recordkeeping. Calif Dent Assoc J 1994;22:30–36.

Legal Considerations of Computer Imaging

13

Edwin J. Zinman, DDS, JD

When used appropriately, computer imaging has the potential to reduce a dentist's exposure to malpractice risk. Based on the clinical experience of practitioners in the field of plastic surgery, there have been no instances of litigation based on the concept of implied warranty.[1] Instead, there have been instances where predictive visualization defused a potentially litigious situation. Properly used, computer imaging can dispel a patient's unrealistic expectations. By visual demonstration, the patient is guided toward realistic treatment goals.

It is important for patients to understand that a computer image represents a treatment goal or direction; a "perfect" result is unlikely.

Anecdotal evidence from other specialties supports the view that computer imaging is detrimental only if it is intentionally used to misrepresent a treatment outcome or to make an unnecessary procedure appear necessary.[2] When used to reasonably illustrate the clinician's expected treatment outcome, imaging is more likely to help avoid legal entanglements with patients. Nevertheless, it is worthwhile to consider the risks a dentist takes with—or without—computer imaging in patient communication.

It is important for patients to understand that a computer image represents a treatment *goal* or *direction;* a "perfect" result is unlikely. A computer can depict changes that are not always precisely predictable or achievable. Individual patient characteristics and the limitations of dental materials and technology may all affect the outcome. In procedures that involve tissue healing, the results may be even less predictable, such as gingival recession around preexisting or planned restorations. Consider consulting a periodontist if gingival esthetic concerns may be affected by gingiva-altering procedures such as subgingival margin placement encroaching near the biologic width space, grafting, or augmentation procedures associated with implant placement. The experiences of cosmetic clinicians, as taught in continuing education courses, can help in the assessment of the probability of esthetic success.

With computer imaging technology, virtually anything may be accomplished. What the patient sees on the monitor, however, is not always achievable clinically. Consequently, never promise more than you can reasonably provide. Articulated study casts are an additional diagnostic aid to determine whether your computer images represent a realistic goal.

Warranty

Unless the dentist promises a particular or precise result, courts will judge esthetic outcomes based on a reasonable patient's expectation, and not an unreasonable, arbitrary, or finicky patient's standard.[3] Informed consent forms are a useful practice aid to help document what the patient was advised. If legal proof ever becomes necessary, informed consent forms document that the dentist made no express warranties guaranteeing a particular result. Form 13-1 is a sample form that can be used to verify the dentist's discussions with the patient. It also helps to prove that esthetic perfection was never promised.

If you intend to give patients a printed image of the proposed esthetic changes, it is advisable to include a disclaimer on each print. Some imaging software will overprint a message such as "Computer simulation—actual results may differ" (Fig 13-1). If you lack encoding software, consider labeling each printed image with such a disclaimer.

A dentist does not ordinarily warrant the success of treatment or even that beneficial results will occur.[4] Nor is it customary for a dentist to promise a cure or achieve any certain result. However, a dentist is liable for breach of warranty if a specific result is promised or guaranteed and the promised result is not achieved. Accordingly, a dentist should promise only to use his or her best efforts to achieve a treatment objective. Avoid promising a particular result such as the patient looking 20 years younger or being able to chew steak again.

For a warranty contract to be legally enforceable, there must be evidence that a written or oral contract existed. A mere therapeutic assurance that the patient will be "all right" does not suffice. Corroborative testimony of witnesses such as the patient's friends, relatives, or dental staff members can constitute express evidence of a warranty contract. Not all of the above items of proof are necessary to transform the tort of professional negligence into a warranty contract guaranteeing a specific result. Rather, courts consider each item of proof in determining whether a dentist made a material representation from which a patient may reasonably expect a particular promised result.

Imaging Informed Consent

In the course of consultations at (practice name), I have been shown or may be shown pictures on an electronic imaging device. I understand that those pictures and alterations of those pictures are solely for the purpose of illustration, discussion, and communication. I understand there may be a difference between the electronic images and my final esthetic result.

I certify my understanding that there is no warranty, expressed or implied, as to my final appearance by the use of these electronically altered images.

Signed:

____________________________ ______________

Patient Date

Signed:

____________________________ ______________

Witness Date

Form 13-1

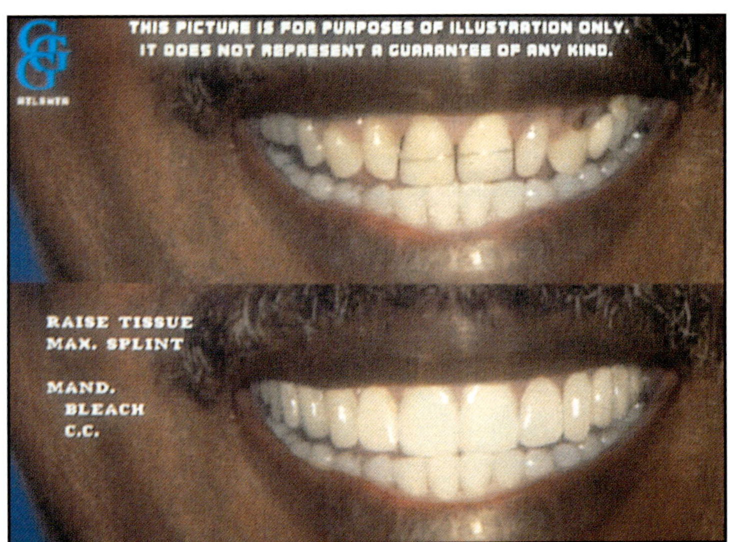

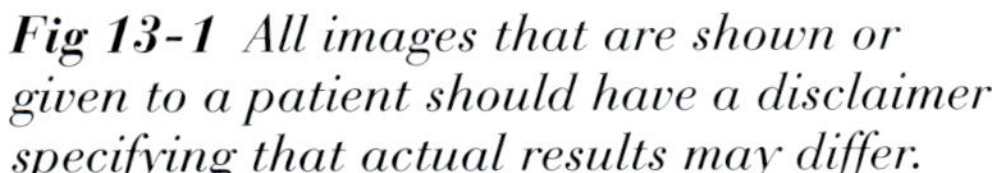

Fig 13-1 *All images that are shown or given to a patient should have a disclaimer specifying that actual results may differ.*

Courts are reluctant to construe treatment discussions between dentist and patient as implying a warranty contract assuring or guaranteeing a favorable result or cure.

Most contracts for dental treatment are oral and simply involve a dentist agreeing to provide professional services rather than a particular result. Accordingly, courts are reluctant to construe treatment discussions between dentist and patient as implying a warranty contract assuring or guaranteeing a favorable result or cure.[5] Notwithstanding, there are court cases upholding warranty contracts for which practitioners were liable for breach of contract for having guaranteed that[6]:

- The patient would be made to look like a model of harmonious perfection.
- Surgery would be performed without pain or scarring, resulting only in hairline scars of minor nature rather than major disfiguring scars.
- Proposed treatment would not worsen the patient's existing condition.
- The patient would be cured within three weeks and could resume business activities.
- 100% function would be restored and an existing impairment eliminated.
- No payment for services would be owed unless the patient was completely satisfied with the end result.
- Dentures would be constructed to the patient's satisfaction and warranted for one year. If, after initial use, the dentures were not functional, the patient's money would be refunded.

Fraudulent Misrepresentation

Proof of fraud or deceit requires proof of an intent to deceive based upon a misrepresentation of proposed treatment and associated hazards. Intentional misrepresentation means that the dentist made false statements with actual knowledge of their falsity, or made false statements without knowing whether they were true or false.

Examples of court-accepted proof of fraud include:

- Accepting any advance payment for treatment that the dentist never intended to perform or never performed
- Misrepresenting unnecessary surgery as necessary
- Misrepresenting the risks of recommended surgery
- Misrepresenting the training or success rate of the treating doctor
- Misrepresenting prognosis when the practitioner lacked knowledge of any reasonably predictive likelihood of complications such as with new or experimental procedures
- Fraudulently concealing poor healing and representing the impaired condition as improving
- Misrepresenting a permanent injury as a transient postoperative problem
- Misrepresenting that surgery had removed all disease

- Inducing the patient to consent to an operation by assuring virtually certain success despite high risks of failure
- Misrepresenting the efficacy of proposed nonsurgical treatment
- Proffering worthless treatment without any curative merits, but instead causing pain, aggravation of the disease, or delay in seeking proper care
- Recommending useless surgery as beneficial
- Concealing the necessity and availability of specialists or second opinion consultation
- Fraudulently concealing a negligent result[7]

Different lighting situations can affect the appearance of esthetic restorations. Thus, even the patient who is pleased with the results of your treatment in your office may later become disillusioned by any subsequent criticism by a spouse or friend. Temporization of restorations before final cementation is advisable to provide the patient an opportunity to evaluate the cosmetic look in different light settings with friends and relatives. For instance, porcelain-fused-to-metal crowns can be temporarily cemented. Then, after a trial period of a week or more, during which the patient can obtain an esthetic stamp of approval from friends or spouse, the patient may be asked to sign a form (Form 13-2) in preparation for final restorations.

Patients can also be asked to sign a release form (Form 13-3) granting permission to use their images for educational or marketing purposes. In most instances, your patient will not be identifiable, although in some cases a full-face photo may be used. Patients who prefer not to have their photos so used may properly decline to sign the release form.

When sending images to your patients, a letter (Form 13-4) may help explain and inform your patient of intended picture usage.

Consent to Final Restorations

Doctor has placed ______________________________,
(name of restoration)

which has functioned in my mouth for ______________________.
(period of time)

I am satisfied with the comfort, fit, and appearance of these restorations and consent to their placement in my mouth with a durable cement, bonding agent, or other appropriate device or material.

Doctor has advised me, and I understand, that a slight variation from the present appearance in some instances may occur after final placement due to the esthetic differences between the temporary and final adhesive materials.

______________________________ ______________
Patient's signature Date

______________________________ ______________
Doctor's signature Date

______________________________ ______________
Witness Date

Form 13-2

Statement of Release

In consideration that my doing so will improve knowledge and further education in the field of dentistry, I hereby consent and agree that the doctors or any person authorized by them may use, reproduce, or otherwise publish photographic or computer illustrations of me in any publications or lecture presentations they may authorize, including the right to use such images in any advertising and promotion of such publication and the dispositions of all rights thereto.

I further agree that I will not assert any claim against any party whatsoever based on the usage of the images or make any claim that the use of the images defames me or constitutes an infringement of my right to privacy or any other right I may enjoy.

I represent that I am 21 years of age or over, and that I have read the foregoing and fully understand the contents thereof and fully agree that I am bound hereby.*

______________________________ _______________
Signature Date

____
Address

______________________________ _______________
Witness Date

**(If the subject of the images is a minor, use the following instead of the last paragraph above.)*

I represent that I am the parent or guardian of _________________________ and that I have read the foregoing and fully understand the contents thereof, and I hereby consent thereto.

______________________________ _______________
Signature Date

____
Address

______________________________ _______________
Witness Date

Form 13-3

Computer Imaging Results

To:

We are enclosing a picture(s) from your computer imaging results. Please note that these photographs are for purposes of illustration only and imply no guarantee whatsoever that your actual surgical or restorative result would or could look this way. Rather it is a beginning point of conversation with your specialist (or with us) to discuss in detail exactly what can be done to improve your appearance.

At times, it is possible to exceed these results and, other times, it is not possible to obtain them. Only your specialist can advise you to what extent he or she can achieve the results indicated here.

We hope that these photographs will be of assistance to you in communication with your specialist (or us).

Most sincerely,

Form 13-4

References

1. *Dorney V. Harris*, (DC Colo) 482 F. Supp. 323.
2. *United States of America v. Rutgard*, 108 F. 3d 1041 (1997).
3. *Rhodes v. Sorokol*, (1993 Tex App. Fort Worth) 846 S.W. 2nd 618; *Willard v. Hagemeister* (1981) 121 Cal. App. 3d, 406, 175 Cal. Rptr. 365.
4. *Perin v. Hayne* (1973, Iowa) 210 N.W. 2nd 609.
5. 11 A.L.R. 4th 748.
6. 61 Am Jur 2d. "Physicians, Surgeons and Other Healers," Section 148; *Broyles v. Brown Engineering Co.* (1963 275 Ala 35, 151 So 2d 767 (dictum); *Guild v. Whitlow* (1924) 162 Ark 108, 257 S.W. 383; *Flowerdew v. Warner* (1965) 90 Idaho 164, 409 P2d 110; *Gault v. Donaldson* (1963) 243 LA 1118, 150 So 2d 35; *Kozan v. Comstock* (1959), CA 5 La, 270 F2d 839, 80 A.L.R. 2d 310 (applying Louisiana law); *Breaux v. Aetna Casualty & Surety Co.* (1967) DC La 272 F. Supp. 668 (applying Louisiana law); *Guilmet v. Campbell* (1971) 385 Mich 57, 188 N.W. 2d 601, 43 A.L.R. 3d 1194; *Vanhoover v. Berghoff* (1887) 90 Mo 487, 3 S.W. 72; *O'Hara v. Wells* (1883) 14 Neb 403, 15 N.W. 722; *Leighton v. Sargent* (1853) 27 N.H. 460; *Grindle v. Rush* (1836) 7 Ohio pt. 2 p. 123; *Kernodle v. Elder* (1909) 23 Okla 743, 102 P. 138; *Shaheen v. Knight* (1957) 11 Pa D & C2d 41, 6 Lycoming R 19; *Yaeger v. Dunnavan* (1946) 26 Wash 2d 559, 174 P2d 755; *Bishop v. Byrne* (1967) D.C. W Va 265 F. Supp. 460; *Rosenblum v. Cherner* (1966, Dist Col App) 219 A. 2d 491, *Burns v. Wanamaker* (1984, App) 281 S.C. 352, 343 S.E. 2nd 27.
7. 83 A.L.R. 2d 114, 4 Proof of Facts 2d 333; 99 A.L.R. 30 303, 43 A.L.R. 3d 1221.

Developing *Technologies*

14

The wide array of choices and the fast pace of development often make the decision to invest in a new, or another, system difficult.

Computer technology is dynamic, and it can be confusing. The wide array of choices and the fast pace of development often make the decision to invest in a new, or another, system difficult. Therefore, it is essential to plan and design carefully with clear and concrete goals and objectives when making decisions to automate your dental practice. While waiting for the next latest and greatest development to appear, you can lose the advantage of providing your patients and yourself with the opportunity for today's optimal dental outcomes using existing technology. You can be sure that many of your professional peers have this technology, and your patients will come to expect it in your practice as well.

While much emphasis has been placed on the marketing value of computer imaging technology, the real benefit is that it improves communication between doctor and patient and makes treatment predictions more concrete. While an imaging system can have a positive economic effect on virtually any practice, justifying the expense, the real value is the contribution to increased excellence in health-care delivery.

What is on the technology horizon? While it's clear that computerized systems will become more powerful, have greater storage capabilities, and become more cost-effective, we can expect to see more development in a number of other areas.

Computerized Diagnostic Systems

Digital radiography

Patients will be particularly appreciative of digital radiography because, in the acquisition of the ordinary periapical film, it reduces radiation exposure by as much as 90% for the patient.[1] This is especially useful in evaluating the marginal integrity of metal-based restorations or the seating of implant abutments where a number of radiographs are required to ensure optimal fit. Often referred to as "filmless radiography," this technology produces a high-quality digitized image that can be electronically manipulated to remove extraneous information, adjust contrast and density, and magnify specific areas of interest without decreasing fidelity. Because the data is in digital form, it can be stored in the automated patient record and transmitted electronically to consulting clinicians if desired.

Voice recognition

While not quite HAL of *2001,* current voice recognition systems are replacing the need for the keyboard or mouse in many situations. For example, physicians can dictate certain medical record reports using key words that have been programmed into an application. In dentistry, voice recognition is part of automated charting systems. During an oral examination, even simple commands such as "open a file" or "store this image" save time and decrease sterile environment risks. The resulting charts, which can be printed, include periodontal, general clinical, occlusal or TMJ, and an assortment of patient medical/dental histories.

Caries detector

A caries detector (Logicon, Trophy, Inc.) can help confirm the probability of caries that cannot be seen definitively on the computerized radiograph. It is a specialized software program that helps to identify the questionable areas and reveal the probability of the questionable area being carious. This can be of enormous value in determining carious lesions at the earliest moment, thus optimizing conservative dental treatment efforts.

Implant software

A presurgical planning software program (such as SIM/Plant, Columbia Scientific, Inc.) allows the dentist to better determine parameters such as implant site, placement, abutment size, canal location, and bone quality analysis for any particular patient. Once a patient has undergone computed tomographic scanning, the information can be transferred to and manipulated by the planning software to prepare a preoperative plan. For example, the placement of multiple root-form implants can be simulated and the implant size and orientation can be modified for optimum position in the patient's bony anatomy.

Occlusal analysis

Once a patient has undergone CT scanning, the information can be transferred to and manipulated by the planning software to prepare a preoperative plan.

Occlusal analysis (T-Scan, Tekscan, Inc.) provides an excellent means of analyzing the functional component of occlusion by recording the timing, location, and intensity of occlusal contacts and displaying the data graphically.[1] The patient bites on a sensor, which is a horseshoe-shaped, double-Mylar film with an electroconductive X–Y grid. The real-time display on the computer monitor shows both the occlusal force and intensity as either a "force snapshot" or a "force movie." The data can be evaluated for treatment implications in esthetic treatment as well as temporomandibular joint examinations, orthodontic evaluation, and prosthetic considerations.

Reflective laser light mapping

Three-dimensional holograms of the head and neck have been available since 1985 from companies pioneering research in this arena. These images, accurate to within a few microns, are captured by a special camera that scans the patient's head and plots more than 250,000 data points. The image obtained can be used to demonstrate potential soft-tissue treatment outcomes in the oral cavity, or the combined result of interspecialty treatment involving possible craniofacial or maxillofacial surgery. Predictive simulations of the effect of situations such as edema or healing and tissue regression can also be considered and/or demonstrated to the patient. The image data is stored in a database and used for analysis and research purposes.

Magnetic resonance imaging

Although MRI is not a new technology, it has new dental applications. As a diagnostic tool, it can be invaluable to patients who have arch deformities. This technology can aid in the simulation of a treatment plan that considers any anomalies of the craniofacial infrastructure for evaluating soft-tissue treatment response probabilities.

Computerized Treatment Systems

CAD/CAM

CAD/CAM will eventually revolutionize the fabrication of fixed prosthodontics, including inlays, laminates, and crowns.

Computer-aided design/computer-aided manufacture will eventually revolutionize the fabrication of fixed prosthodontics, including inlays, laminates, and crowns. For example, it is possible to produce a digital "impression" of a tooth preparation with a computer imaging technique; a reflective powder is applied to the prepared tooth surface and a digital camera scans the preparation, quantifying the reflected light by measuring and correlating thousands of data points. The resulting three-dimensional image is used by a computer-controlled lathe to carve a restoration to exact specifications of mesial-distal diameter, height, and fit. As this technology is enhanced and refined, it will provide for relatively immediate and accurate restorative capabilities. Orthopedic surgeons have used similar applications to custom design and manufacture hip joints during replacement surgery.

Another approach to CAD/CAM is the remote CAM process (Procera, Nobel Biocare), which produces extremely strong titanium or all-ceramic cores for crowns and bridges. The prepared model (die) is scanned by a device in the dental office, the information is transferred to a PC data file, and it is then electronically transmitted to a manufacturing location in Sweden. There, the core is processed in densely sintered aluminum oxide. The result is shipped to the dental office location within four days, a manufacture time frame that approximates the conventionally constructed restoration. Further, the advantage of Procera, in addition to the increased strength of the core, is that the titanium construction is veneered with a special porcelain to give strong bonding, high wear resistance, and optimum esthetics.

Laser technology

Although lasers have been used in dentistry in one form or another during the last decade, expect a resurgence of their use. A new diode laser that is much smaller and more mobile than previous models works well for multi-operatory environments. Argon lasers, in either water- or air-cooled models, can be centrally installed with individual wands and placed and used as conveniently as the high-speed handpiece in each dental unit. The advent of lasers that treat hard tissues offer continuing progress in painless and conservative restorative dentistry.

Bleaching with laser technology. For laser bleaching, the argon laser curing light is used, either by itself or in combination with other lasers. It, along with most other forms of in-office and matrix bleaching, can be an effective means for lightening yellow and even some brown and gray stained teeth.

Air-abrasive technology

Air-abrasive technology may represent the quest for conservative dentistry in its highest form. Rather than ignoring a darkly stained pit or fissure, or using the traditional high-speed handpiece method to remove it, the dentist can use air-abrasive technology to gently spray away the stain and the underlying organic plug with alpha alumina particles.[2] If caries, or "veins of decay," are present, they can be seen either directly or in conjunction with the intraoral camera. The caries can usually be removed with the air-abrasive without removing larger amounts of sound tooth structure required by the conventional handpiece.

Air-abrasive instrumentation generates little heat compared to high-speed rotary instrumentation, and is therefore kinder to the pulp. This reduction of temperature elevation, along with the elimination of bone-conducted noise and vibration, means that most air-abrasive procedures can be performed without anesthesia. Further, the alpha alumina particles increase the surface area of the tooth, which, when combined with conventional etching procedures, produces a stronger mechanism for retaining sealants and/or composite restorations.[3] This technology is also valuable for the repair of marginal defects, as well as all types of composite resin or ceramic restorations.[2]

Informed Choices

Many dentists feel that they can never know enough about computer technology to make an informed choice. There are many available sources that can get you started in the right direction. You may want to consider a book or course that is designed specifically for analyzing dental business and clinical systems, or a consultant who can provide varying levels of assistance to educate you sufficiently. You can gain a surprising amount of knowledge with just a little time and effort. It bears repeating that careful systems analysis and design are key to successfully choosing the technology that best supports the particular needs of your dental practice.

For those of you who object to the cost and learning curve associated with computerizing the clinical activities in your practice, be aware of the consequences. Your patients may silently tell you that you should have made that investment by seeking services such as imaging in another dental office. The forward-thinking dentist will continue to adapt technology to areas beyond traditional practice management functions and will embrace the new and innovative clinical applications. While not every new technology will be appropriate for every practice, selective choices will keep your practice progressive and dynamic. New technology can energize your day-to-day activities with innovative diagnostic and treatment procedures, giving you greater personal and professional satisfaction.

References

1. Goldstein RE, Miller MC. High technology in esthetic dentistry. Curr Opin Cosmet Dent 1993, 5–11.
2. Goldstein RE, Parkins FM. Using air-abrasive technology to diagnose and restore pit and fissure caries. JADA 1995; 126:761–766.
3. Goldstein RE, Parkins FM. Air-abrasive technology: its new role in restorative dentistry. JADA 1994; 125:551–557.

15 Some Common *Questions* About Computer Imaging Systems

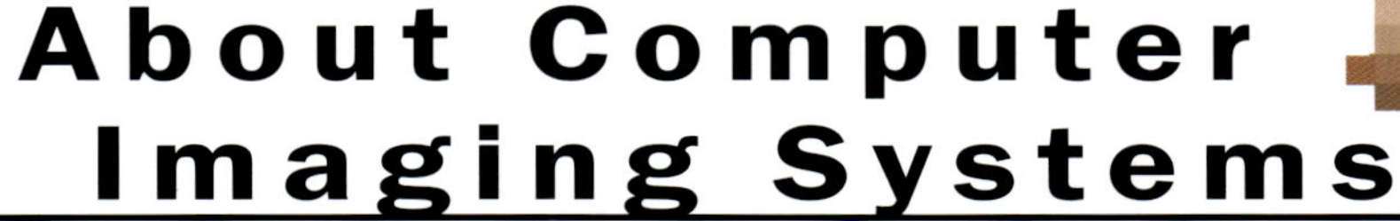

Q ***How can I determine the best system for my needs?***

A Computer systems are designed to do a multitude of tasks. Therefore, you may want or expect the computer you purchase for dental imaging to also handle your practice management and billing. A rule of thumb is that you try to buy more computer than you need now. The difference in price between the minimum system you need and the next step up is usually quite small. Besides, it's virtually assured that you will regret it later if you skimp now. This is more a reflection of current limitations in the state of the art than anything else. Although some aggressive, futuristic plans are being designed at this writing, some or many of the technologies you will be using in the future are not designed to work together well just now. Even if they were designed to interface with one another, the combined load could overwhelm current systems because of their limited processing power and available memory.

It may seem ridiculous to call today's technology "limited," but read this chapter in three years and you'll see what we mean. Reduced instruction set computer (RISC) systems, already available, significantly increase available computer power. In the future, appropriately powered systems designs with ample memory will be able to support the full array of clinical and business applications. Today, a practical architecture for an integrated practice management/ clinical environment should focus on the consolidation of database information. One approach would be the use of a RISC-based server that drives a network of integrated workstations and collects information in a relational database format.

Although some manufacturers are touting systems that do everything, they are not as appropriately integrated as they can or should be and the compromises are obvious. The fascinating yet frustrating aspect of this discourse is the geometric progression in technological advancement. In the course of writing this text, many changes in technology have occurred, necessitating numerous rewrites. So, take this advice in context and look for updates from time to time.

In any event, no matter how technology advances, some of the best advice you can get will come from your peers. If a salesperson calls on you, request a list of clients and call them. Don't be shy about asking questions. What are they doing with their system? Does it do everything they wanted it to? If not, what's missing? Are they satisfied with its speed? The technical support? Training? Documentation? Did the vendor provide tutorial materials or only reference materials?

What the salesperson won't tell you, your peers may. You want a dependable system that is easy to use, one with excellent training provided by the vendor. A system with minimal training for you and your staff and questionable credentials is no bargain if it fails to satisfy your needs after you buy it and the vendor is nowhere to be found. Technical considerations aside, these issues of human interaction are much more important than once thought, making the chemistry of the relationship between you and your vendor a vital factor in choosing the right system.

Q *Are there any major differences between systems?*

A The short answer is no, but computers are a complex subject, and different systems have different features.

Your first consideration will likely be whether you want an IBM (or IBM-compatible) system or a Macintosh (Apple). These two very popular computer systems have traditionally been as different as day and night. However, with the joint venture activities launched between IBM and Apple, as well as ongoing efforts to improve system interface and file interchangeability, the differences between IBM and Mac systems will become less important.

In the past, the IBM or compatible system used an operating system—usually Microsoft Corporation's Disk Operating System (MS-DOS)—that was somewhat intimidating to the novice user. This was largely tolerated because the system could be mastered easily enough with a little determination. Also important was the clout of IBM and its commitment to MS-DOS, which fostered the development of literally millions of IBM PCs or compatible computers in use today. IBM's system became, therefore, a de facto standard. Users had no trouble finding competent personnel to operate their computers, and a large selection of applications software was available.

The Macintosh computer system, on the other hand, was marketed as "the computer for the rest of us" to emphasize that its interface, or operating system, is simple, intuitive, and highly graphical. In other words, the Mac performs complex operations the way you think, not according to strict "computerese." It consequently enjoyed a period of increasing popularity in business, although that has been eroded by the introduction of Microsoft Windows and IBM's OS/2 operating system. Still, the Macintosh has a substantial software library to choose from. One disadvantage to the Macintosh is that traditionally it has been significantly more expensive than a similarly configured IBM or compatible computer system. The cost differential is attributable to market forces: Macintosh clones have become available only recently, while there are literally hundreds of competing companies making IBM clones.

Your needs should determine which system you buy. If the software or applications programs you want are available for both IBM and Macintosh, try both systems at a dealer, talk with your peers about the pros and cons of each, and then decide. Both systems are excellent.

What to evaluate in an operating system

1. Easy to use (Windows based)
2. Price
3. Image resolution
   - Clear/bright
   - Little or no distortion
   - Not a reversed image
   - True colors
4. Memory capacity/speed
5. Warranty/technical support/loaners
6. Open architecture
7. Printer/VCR
8. Compact/moveable
9. Sterility
10. Master system with independent stations
11. Nonfocus, wide depth of field
12. One tooth or a full arch, all areas
13. Combined system, with intraoral and extraoral imaging
14. Small, comfortable swivel handpiece
15. Help screen/video tutorial
16. Nonfogging lens
17. Quiet

Aside from the issue of what type of system to choose, you must also decide whether you want a single-user or a multi-user system. Simply put, the single-user system is designed to be used by one person at a time. The multi-user system is configured with different workstations, enabling a number of people to work and exchange information concurrently. If your needs are strictly imaging, a single-user system is probably sufficient for that purpose. Likewise, if your billing and practice management can be done on one system, there is no reason to purchase an extensive network of multi-user computers. Obviously, the more people who can access or use a computer system, the more expensive and complex that system will be. But it will also be more versatile and useful, potentially, and is justified if you need multi-user capabilities.

Q *Should I lease or buy outright?*

A This is a question for your accountant. Tax laws change and the advantages of leasing over purchasing can vary greatly, depending on your situation. Only in consultation with your accountant can you consider the particulars of a wide range of factors—including your business, your balance sheet, and your banking relationships—that underlie this decision. However, the following discussion should provide you with some general background.

A common misconception is that you can lease a system for a short period of time to determine whether it will meet your needs. However, you will probably find that a lease is just as much of a commitment as an outright purchase and that short-term leases typically carry a very high premium for the option of returning the equipment after only a few months. Leasing also has little to do with your ability to upgrade your system as technology advances. While an appropriately negotiated lease can *sometimes* provide for the ability to upgrade your system, do the following: work with a company that has an established record of keeping its customers' systems current, and do not view a short-term lease as an opportunity to "test drive" a system.

If you are considering a system for dental imaging, leasing could be an advantage—but it may not be a significant one. Interest rates determine lease factors, and as volatile as rates have been over the last few years, locking in a leased system at a good price might be harder than you think. An advantage to purchasing is that simple-interest loans from your banker almost always carry a lower interest rate and offer greater flexibility if you decide to pay off your loan early. Moreover, you can treat part of the purchase cost as services and training, and write off 100% of that cost in the first year. Another advantage is that you may save the cost of sales tax if you purchase from an out-of-state vendor and your state does not require reporting such purchases. If you lease, you will definitely pay sales tax or use tax, regardless of where you or your computer vendor reside, because you are dealing with a leasing company chartered to do business in your state; the leasing company buys a system from the vendor, and you, in essence, reimburse the leasing company.

The primary advantages of leasing are convenience and what has been referred to as "off balance sheet financing." In the past, leases didn't appear on the balance sheet in the same way a bank loan would. Leasing the majority of your capitalized equipment therefore allowed you to have a great deal of equipment without encumbering your balance sheet. Today, however, a properly audited balance sheet will reflect leases as existing obligations. Still, you have only a certain amount of credit available through your local banker no matter how successful you may be. Leasing is a way to keep your line of credit available for operational needs, remodeling, and other costs of business.

Two Types of Leases

If you are considering a lease, there are two basic types to compare. One is called a "true lease" and is also known as a "guideline lease" or a "tax lease." This type of lease is tailored to tax laws and is the only type that meets the Internal Revenue Service definition of a lease. The true lease is characterized by a lease term that matches IRS depreciation schedules for the type of equipment being leased. It typically has no preset purchase option at the end of the lease, and you will usually pay your first and last months' payments at the inception of the lease. When the term ends, you may either purchase the equipment for its fair market value or return it to the leasing company.

Leasing is a way to keep your line of credit available for operational needs, remodeling, and other costs of business.

The second type of lease is regarded by tax accountants as a "conditional purchase agreement." It looks like a lease but may or may not require up-front cash and almost always has a prearranged purchase option at the end of the lease term. Two commonly used purchase options are the 10% buyout, in which you can purchase the equipment at the end of the lease for 10% of the system's initial purchase price; and the $1 buyout, also known as an "abandonment lease," in which you acquire title to the equipment for $1 at the end of the lease.

Frankly, there is little difference between these options. The best way to analyze the variants is to add the cash outlay at inception plus the cost of ownership at the end of the lease to the total cost of the monthly payments. You will probably find little net difference in the final figures. Given that, you will probably opt for the 10% buyout over the $1 buyout for two important reasons. First, you will be paying for the ownership option in future dollars that will surely be less valuable than current dollars. Second, you will end up paying interest on that 10% over the life of the contract if you opt instead for the $1 buyout. And finally, in five years you may want to make big changes that don't include the equipment you lease today. For example, we have found high technology in our office, particularly our extraoral imaging system, to be productive and profitable. In five years, we may want to invest in state-of-the-art technology that may or may not include our current components.

In any event, keep in mind that there may be tax advantages to using one type of lease over another; but again, that depends on your individual situation and can be determined by your tax accountant.

Buying outright may save you some money, since lease arrangements tie you to a specific computer model and vendor. For example, IBM makes a good personal computer that might sell for $2,900, while a virtually identical system from Compaq Computers sells for $2,000. The computers are comparable in features and performance. Yet, if you are tied to a lease, you may get the IBM system, although the less expensive and highly rated Compaq could meet your needs equally well.

Regardless of how you acquire your imaging system, make sure you have a firm, reliable commitment for service and training on the equipment. Your imaging computer can be one of the most important assets you've ever added to your practice. It is much more than just a "revenue generator." It can be your electronic photography center, patient records archival system, patient communications center, and your baseline system for treatment planning. However, if it is out of order, or your staff doesn't know how to take advantage of its features, it becomes nothing more than an expensive, high-tech boat anchor!

Q *I've decided to acquire an imaging system. What now?*

A Once you have made a decision to acquire an imaging system, you need to collect information. Professional consultants use a Request for Proposal (RFP) or Request for Information (RFI) form. This is a structured document that details all of the information you should collect from each vendor and analyze for appropriateness for your individual needs. Whether you purchase this document or develop your own, the basic RFP/RFI should request the information described at the top of the next page.

Provide the RFP/RFI to each vendor and require them to answer it in your format. Do not allow them to submit only their own standardized information package, because you will then have the enormous task of organizing, analyzing, and comparing the information from all vendors. Give a firm, but reasonable, due date and include a statement that the answers supplied by the vendor will become part of your contract for acquiring the system.

Information to obtain from potential vendors

- Vendor corporate history, including current financial status, location, and size of company
- Complete listing of clients, including contact names and numbers
- Detailed list of all software and hardware components of the proposed system
- A section detailing the data fields you require
- A section detailing the communications and integration capabilities you require
- Proposed length of system usefulness, given the size and growth pattern of your practice
- Upgrade pathway of the proposed system
- Complete breakdown of all software, hardware, training, support, and documentation costs
- Amount and location of training (eg, on-site or training facility)
- Number of *dedicated* trainers and support personnel (ie, *not* the salesman)
- Cost and availability of ongoing support
- Information on who provides the support (hardware and software) and toll-free number, if available
- Warranties that come with the system
- Policy for software enhancements (cost and availability)
- Financial arrangements offered by the vendor

After careful analysis of the RFP/RFI, you should be able to determine the two or three vendors that will best meet your needs. Your next step should be to contact a random selection of clients to inquire about their experience with the system and the vendor. Prepare a list of standardized questions to ask each of them. For example, you might ask if the software and hardware work as expected, if the support and training are adequate, or how the vendor reacts to problem situations. It may also be wise to visit one or more actual client sites to review the system in operation. This may be done with or without the vendor representative present.

Finally, keep in mind that every point of your negotiations and expectations should be expressed in a *written* contract. If you are promised that your new imaging system will work seamlessly with your existing business management system, make it a contract-dependent issue. If this is the first time that your imaging vendor is attempting to integrate with the business system vendor, and you agree to be the first live site (beta site), define specifically what is and what is not acceptable.

Also, beware of software, or software components, computations, data fields, and, especially, communications, that are "in development." Until you see it work, consider it vaporware. And contractually arrange to pay for it accordingly.

This process may seem laborious, but it is a proven method for system selection. You are more likely to have a system that meets your needs now and in the future if you give careful attention to the selection process.

Q *Should I expect a company to update my system?*

A Any computer system or software applications package comes with a warranty registration card, which should be filled out and returned to the manufacturer so that you will be informed about product changes, enhancements, and updates. The decision of whether to act on that information and update a system or applications package is yours. While it is unusual for companies to automatically upgrade their systems, some may have this type of policy.

More often than not, you will have to pay for the updated version of the product. As a rule, an update that enhances an existing feature of the program may be provided at no charge or at a minimal charge; changes that add significant new capabilities carry a higher price tag. Usually, companies will provide upgrades free of charge within a certain time period after you purchase your system. That period can range from 90 days to a year.

It has been our experience that upgrades usually add value to the applications program or product and should be considered on their individual merits.

Q *Do I need a printer?*

A Yes, if you intend to give your patients a tangible record of your planned result. A printer will also allow you to communicate more effectively with your laboratory by providing useful visual information that can help you and the lab technician confer on the case and plan changes.

A printer also provides a good photographic record to include in your patient's file. Finally, a print-out of your patient's treatment plan can be a real help in the event that your computer images are erased or something happens to your disk.

Q

Should my patient watch me or the imaging technician work?

A

There are good arguments for and against having the patients present, but we generally find it helpful to include the patient in an interactive session with the imaging system. Inviting patients to participate gives them the opportunity to offer their input while you manipulate their image. And research has shown that such patient involvement can help produce more successful results.[1] Patients can quickly respond to what they do or do not like, giving you more information on which to base your suggestions, so that together you can settle on a mutually agreeable plan.

This period of "co-diagnosis" helps patients understand what will and will not work so they can accept the results. It is also helpful in dispelling unrealistic expectations. We have often interviewed patients whose hopes for how the finished case will look are unachievable. Their view is not based on how they actually appear, but on how they *wish* they appeared. Interactive imaging is the only way we have found to uncover these troublesome misconceptions and convert a potentially litigious patient to one who is happy and enthusiastic posttreatment. In extreme instances, the imaging system identifies the patient who will never be satisfied, regardless of the final result. In such cases, we are obliged to refuse treatment, knowing that the patient's problem is not related to dental health or esthetics.

Be aware that there can be some drawbacks to having the patient watch while you image proposed changes. For example, patients may become bored if the process takes too long. Also, in trying out different approaches to a patient's problem, you may make changes that can appear comical and just plain wrong for your patient. You may make the teeth too long, too yellow, too white, or experiment with a new hairstyle that does nothing to flatter the patient's features. Patients may feel self-conscious watching these trials. Therefore, if you sense that an individual patient may be too sensitive to work with you comfortably, it may be advisable to ask the patient to come back at a later date to view your proposals. This will give you an opportunity to study the patient's face and smile in privacy and plan improvements. Admittedly, these instances are rare and preempt the opportunity for the patient to participate, so don't make this decision on the patient's behalf without careful consideration.

Finally, if patients watch you work, they may see you try changes that prove impossible to achieve. Since many users of imaging systems will delegate the task of patient imaging to an assistant or hygienist, it is important that you as the clinician review proposed changes to ascertain whether you can deliver the results shown. In any event, the notion that the computer will image results that cannot be achieved and thus create a malpractice risk is not justified. Handled properly, the system will only illustrate changes you feel confident you can achieve.

As an experienced clinician, you form an image in your head of how the final result will appear. You base that image on your training, experience, and skill. Most likely, your results are generally consistent with that initial image you create in your mind. The imaging system is merely a means to get that image from your head and onto the computer screen so you can share your vision more clearly with your patient.

In short, you will need to assess each patient individually before deciding whether to image changes with or without the patient's participation. Some patients will want to be part of the process. Others will be on a tight timetable and will want to see your interpretation only when you are finished. Be flexible. We have found that in most circumstances, patients enjoy and are intrigued with the computer imaging process, and their input can be beneficial.

Q ***Should I suggest other changes, like a different hairstyle or plastic surgery?***

A This depends on each patient's attitude toward your esthetic input. Some patients will appreciate all you do for them, while others will consider your suggesting a new hairstyle or facial surgery insulting. So the first rule is, *know your patient*. One approach is to let your patient know what your computer program is capable of doing and let the patient's reactions be your guide. For instance, you might say, "If you have ever wanted to see how you would look as a blond (brunette or redhead) or with a 'pug' nose, now is the time to do it!" This should be said in a friendly, almost jovial way, so that it will not be taken as an insult.

If you feel your patient will receive your suggestions in the right spirit, create a third or fourth image. The screen can be split into thirds as shown below.

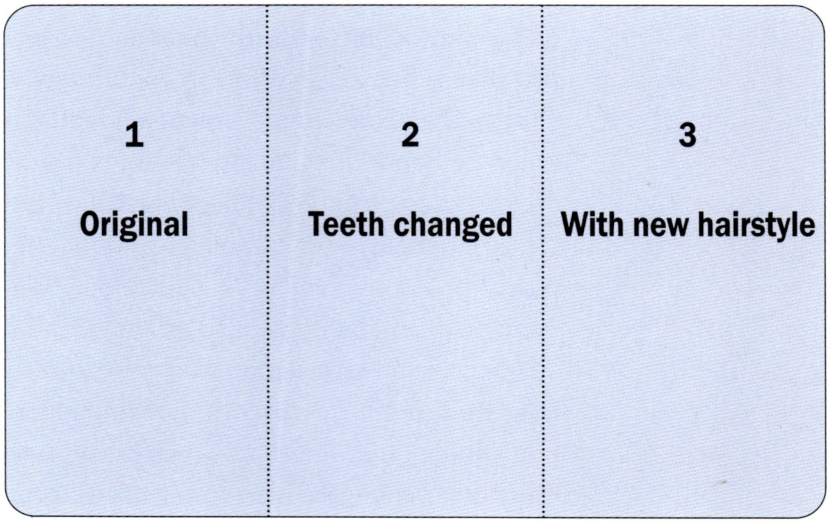

1	2	3
Original	**Teeth changed**	**With new hairstyle**

 *Is it possible to spend too much time altering an image?*

 Yes and no. Many people can visualize the intended results quickly and will need to see only a preliminary mock-up on the screen before giving their approval. You can tell this patient before you start, "Let me know when you're satisfied with the changes, and then we can talk more about the plan." This approach lets you show the patient step-by-step what you'd recommend. Again, you need to know your patient. Sometimes you can spend too long on this or say too much!

On the other hand, some patients will need to see a detailed image of what you intend to do for them. Then you will probably want to make all of your alterations, blend them, and get the best image possible before presenting it to your patient.

Since you will be showing your patient with a new, different smile or facial result, it may take time before your patient feels comfortable with a totally new look. Having time to digest the print-out with one's spouse, and friends and family, may be just what he or she needs to feel comfortable enough to proceed. Be supportive and understanding of these patients. Realize that their indecision may be their decision, and if it is, you will be better-off knowing that before, rather than after (possibly extensive) therapy. No one wants an esthetic failure. Computer imaging can be the best technology to help you prevent an esthetic failure.

Reference

1. Rosenthal L, Pleasure M, Lefer L. Patient reaction to denture esthetics. J Dent Med 1964;19:103.

Index

Page references followed by "f" denote figures.

A

B

C

L

M

N

O

P

Q

R